DIETS SUCK!

READ WHAT PEOPLE ARE SAYING

"*DIETS SUCK!* is a must-have if you're ready to take control of your health. I hope you enjoy this book as much as I have."

—Keith Ferrazzi, NY Times Bestselling Author of *Never Eat Alone* and *Who's Got Your Back*

"If you're in the market for a great book on how to boost your health and lose weight naturally this year, all while being incredibly inspired, this is a must-read."

—Dr. Michael Dow, Author, Psychotherapist, Host of TLC's *Freaky Eaters*

"*DIETS SUCK!* is a wonderful, easy-to-read book that gives you the 'Principles' for successful long-term weight loss."

—Russell Cleveland, Author of *Finding Midas: Investing in Entrepreneurial CEOs with the Golden Touch;* Financial Executive, RENN Capital Group

"Wow! Stephen's enthusiasm, expertise, and wit come through like a lighthouse in the fog and make this a fun book about how to lose weight. You'll cheer for Audrey as the story unfolds, and you'll learn her secrets to losing weight and becoming healthy."

—Todd Ordal, Former Division President Kinko's; Certified Management Consultant

"It is with great admiration and pride that I enthusiastically recommend you read on and pay attention to what Stephen has to say in this book, *DIETS SUCK!* His message has changed my life and the lives of so many others already. I am sure it can do the same for you too."

—Andrew M. Rosenthal, M.D., Harvard Medical School

"*DIETS SUCK!* is a refreshing take on an important topic. Stephen and Sue are able to take a normally difficult topic and inspire through story. I recommend this for anyone who wants to take ownership of their health and fitness."

—Dr. Mark Goulston, Psychiatrist and NY Times Bestselling Author

---

"Finally! A book that gives advice in a wonderfully enjoyable format. Through the parables presented in *DIETS SUCK!* I was able to not only learn but be inspired and then empowered. I highly recommend this book to anyone looking to take control of the choices in their life."

—Frances Cole Jones, Media Coach and Bestselling Author of *How to Wow* and *The Wow Factor.*

"As a person who has been constantly on 'diets' and trying to keep myself 'forever young,' this is the best book I have read! Stephen Adele's writing is crystal clear, succinct, and spot on. I highly recommend this to anyone who is tired of dieting and ready for lasting results. It has helped me and my family in all endeavors."

—W. Terrance Schreier, Managing Director, Transition Partners LTD, and Former General Counsel to the Kansas City Royals MLB

"I've been close friends with Stephen Adele for many years, and he is genuinely passionate about helping people reach their fitness and wellness goals. He accomplishes this without gimmicks but with life lessons everyday people can apply to help fuel their own personal transformations. *DIETS SUCK!* is a must-read for anyone looking to jump start their journey to a life of health and wellness."

—Eric Hillman, CEO, Europa Sports Products

"Stephen Adele's book *DIETS SUCK!* is a very practical, true-to-life slap in the face as to the reality of how we live our lives and how ineffective and ridiculous the aspect of 'dieting' truly is. This book is incredibly thought-provoking because it is a non-fictional account of one person's ongoing struggle turned into a battle easily won with motivation, dedication, and commitment. The book will make you smile and laugh, but can also make you cry when one actually weighs in on how close it cuts to the quick for most of us."

—Darryn Willoughby, Ph.D., FACSM, FISSN, CSCS, CISSN, Department of Health, Human Performance, and Recreation, Baylor University

---

"As a physician, I know firsthand that 'diets' can be as unhealthy as healthy. This book successfully approaches a person's lifestyle and creates real results. I recommend *DIETS SUCK!* for anyone wanting to be a better version of this self. Doctors orders!"

—Dr. Sanjay Jain, M.D., MBA, "The Balance Guy," International Speaker and Author

---

"DIETS *do* SUCK! I've been there myself; I found the stories in this book not only informative but equally inspiring. A terrific read!"

—Gina Rudan, Author, Thought Leader, and Mother of Two

"The title says it all. This is an advice book that delivers realistic solutions in a clear language that's perfect for those who have despaired after trying fad diets that never work."

—Jim Schmaltz, Editor-in-Chief of *Muscle & Body* and Editorial Director of *Physique 3D* Magazines

---

"*DIETS SUCK!* is more than a book about diets. It's about self-empowerment and triumph in today's harsh society. It eloquently retells the stories of real people who ultimately take control of their lives emotionally, mentally, and physically. There's no denying that people will relate to Audrey's journey and be inspired to make real, sustainable changes in their everyday routines. In fact, I couldn't help but have my own 'Satori' moment while reading these pages. It just makes sense."

—Kerrie Lee Brown, former Editor-in-Chief of *Oxygen* Women's Fitness Magazine, Founding Editor of *American Health & Fitness*, and VP, STOTT PILATES®

Author's Disclaimer about the Characters and Setting of this Book

The stories surrounding the main character found in this book are based on the astoundingly true physical and mental transformation of Andrea Clem. The story line and setting presented here are based on actual events. Andrea discovered the Lessons found in this book through a variety of different means, but not all necessarily in direct meetings with me (as depicted by my character in the story). Yet she ultimately learned and, more importantly, applied the Lessons to her life, and the end results can be seen not only in her inspiring before and after photos but also in virtually every aspect of her life. The other "success stories" found throughout the book are also completely true, their names are not changed, and their photos are un-retouched. iSatori is a real company, and I am the founder and CEO. You can learn more about us at iSatori.com or meet me online at Facebook.com/StephenAdele.

DIETS SUCK!

A Remarkably Inspiring Story of
Physical & Emotional Transformation

BY STEPHEN ADELÉ
with Sue Mosebar

IRON WARRIOR MEDIA, GOLDEN, CO

Published by
Iron Warrior Media
Golden, CO

Publisher's Cataloging-in-Publication Data
Adelé, Stephen, 1971-

Diets suck! : a remarkably inspiring story of physical and emotional transformation /
by Stephen Adelé with Sue Mosebar. – Golden, CO : Iron Warrior Media, 2014.

p. ; cm.

ISBN13: 978-0-9860698-0-2

1. Weight loss. 2. Health. 3. Exercise. I. Title. II. Mosebar, Sue.

RM222.2.A34 2014
613.25—dc23   2013952239

FIRST EDITION

Project coordination by Jenkins Group, Inc.
www.BookPublishing.com

Interior design by Brian Harvat

Printed in the United States of America
18 17 16 15 14 • 5 4 3 2 1

This book is dedicated to all those transformational "success stories" who have inspired us to share this story; and those who will soon walk in your footsteps.

CONTENTS

THE MODEL

THE EXTRAS (Must-Read Addendums)

FOREWORD

It was a day I will never forget and a day that changed my life forever.

Two and a half years ago, I discovered I had cancer. It was quite by accident and came as a complete shock. See, I am a board-certified diagnostic radiologist, so you can imagine my dismay the night I detected two malignant tumors in my own body as I read my CT scan. I couldn't believe what I was seeing. I had diagnosed my own potentially fatal cancer. As I stared at the scan images, I quickly realized, in that very moment, *everything* in my life was about to change, forever.

As a Harvard-educated physician, with residency training at Harvard's Brigham Hospital and Columbia-Presbyterian Medical Center, and a fellowship at Cornell–New York Hospital, I have spent over 30 years diagnosing illness and delivering news to patients. Sometimes the news was heartbreaking, and sometimes the news was uplifting. But it was always news about *other* people. This time, it was about me.

Whether or not my eating habits, stress, or other approaches to life had anything to do with me getting cancer, I'll never know. Maybe it was just bad luck. But what I do know is I was about to change the way I ate, the way I lived, and how I interacted with my family and friends from that day forward.

I soon began to educate myself about nutrition and exercise and stress reduction. But I also knew a "prescription for health" emphasizing these important factors wasn't the total answer. I soon realized there were many other very important and powerful ways to improve health and life that went beyond nutrition and exercise.

One day, by chance, I met Mr. Stephen Adelé. This young man surprised me by something he said about nutrition and health. He believed when it came to improving our health, our performance, and our appearance, diets don't work. He was adamant that diets fail *us all.* Not that we fail diets, but that diets fail us. This statement was novel and thought provoking. As I got to know Stephen better, I discovered his deep and genuine passion for helping individuals from all walks of life change their habits and lifestyle to improve the way they look and feel.

Soon thereafter, I attended a conference in New York, where Stephen was making a presentation. We scheduled a short meeting to follow, and that short meeting turned into several hours of meaningful conversation. I was struck by how knowledgeable and caring Stephen was. It was clear this young man had something important to say. I took his advice to heart. He has a unique approach to modifying one's outlook to make positive lifestyle changes geared to immediate and long-lasting improvements in well-being.

Two and a half years later, with hard work, an uphill battle, and inspiration from Stephen, I am living life healthier and happier than ever before. My views on life have definitely changed, and despite everything that has happened, I maintain a positive outlook.

So it is with great admiration and pride that I enthusiastically recommend you read on and pay attention to what Stephen has to say in this book. His message has changed my life and the lives of so many others already. I am sure it can do the same for you too.

Yours in health and spirit,

Andrew M. Rosenthal, M.D.
Harvard Medical School
Class of 1975

THE STORY

THE DAY

Audrey Smith had no idea today would be *the day* that would change her life forever.

After 34 years of living life in the shadows of her siblings, struggling with her body weight—from elementary school through torturous teenage years and on into adulthood after having two children—Audrey's self-image was in the dumps.

Trying diet after diet… From crazy fad diets… to calorie and point-counting systems… to dangerous diet pills, *Audrey had tried it all,* with little to no success. Despite countless attempts, her weight had continued to creep up over the years, and her health was slowly deteriorating with it. She was left with feelings of inadequacy and hopelessness, and a physical appearance she was not proud of. On top of that, she felt like she was letting herself, and her family, down.

But today that would all change, *forever*. What Audrey didn't know was how her journey to regain her body and life would surprisingly unfold.

INTRODUCTION

Our greatest struggle is within ourselves.

Whatever sense we have that we *know* something, or have *the* answer, often becomes the barrier to our learning. And, without question, limits our ability to improve ourselves. I've found this especially true when it comes to improving the way we look and feel.

Over the years, my experiences have led me to believe there is something fundamentally wrong with our approach to changing our physical appearance. Otherwise, we wouldn't be the most obese nation in the civilized world. Simply persuading people to eat less, exercise more—and when that doesn't work fast enough, resort to diet drugs or stomach surgeries—isn't working. Worse, resorting to fad diets could be the most destructive contributor of all.

Let's face it—*Diets Suck!*

Think about it. Every diet has a starting point and an ending point. Whether it's seven days or three months, you have to endure it. Struggle, from day to day, to find the willpower to keep going. Deprive yourself. In some cases, starve yourself. *And for what?* Maybe a temporary "quick-fix"—losing 5 or 10 or 15 pounds. Only to regain it all back, once you stop the diet, usually to put on a few extra pounds for good measure.

Every year, over 60% of us will start some sort of fad diet in the hope of losing weight. To make matters worse, most people will try up to three or four diets in a single year. This vicious cycle, unfortunately, repeats itself year after year.

Where does the madness stop? Well, I am here to tell you, my friend, it stops right here. Right now.

No more crazy dieting. No more starving yourself. No more eating frozen, prepared foods. No more visits to the nearby weight-loss clinic. And, no more resorting to "magic pills."

Not in this book.

Because, in my opinion, and from what I've witnessed over the years, **diets don't work.** Once I learned to fully embrace this concept, and the more I worked with people from all walks of life to create rapid and lasting physical changes, the more I have become convinced this is true.

In other words, *we* don't fail: the "diets" we follow fail *us*. Reason is, they are inherently counterproductive to our natural way of living. That is, we are human beings, designed by our Great Creator to eat. We love food. I know I do. And I'm sure you do too. And there is no reason we should deprive ourselves of food. But that is not to say all foods are created equal. *Far from it.*

If you think about it, for all the attention nutrition and eating "healthy" has received over the years from scholars, coaches, teachers, the media, and through the sensationalizing of fad diets, learning how to *eat smarter* is as elusive as it has ever been for most people.

See, unlike most other things in our lives, one thing we can control is our bodies and what we put *into* them and what we do *with* them, and consequently, our health and well-being. But like so many other aspects of life, changing the way you look—improving your physical appearance—comes down to practicing a very simple, small set of behaviors. But as I have unfortunately experienced with most people, they're not always as easily put into practice day after day.

After devoting the last 20 years of my life to working closely with thousands upon thousands of clients, in guiding them to transform their physical appearances, I've studied—*very carefully*—each and every one. Learned their habits, both good *and* bad. And over time, I've learned what works, and equally important, what doesn't.

During this time, I've learned that the *truly successful* weight-loss transformations come only for those people who overcome the all-too-human behavioral pitfalls that can derail their desire to eat smarter and breed the dreadful on-again-off-again dieting tendencies, or *eating "dumb,"* as I call them.

Along the way, I invested countless hours studying the history of the human diet—from our ancient ancestors in Biblical times to our typical modern day diet. I also spent *many* late nights reading scientific abstracts and published articles on the science of weight loss and how the biochemistry of food affects our bodies.

And through this effort, I was able to come away with a very clear set of "core" principles. Seven in fact. Some of which were pretty startling. As it turned out, these principles applied to more than just eating smart. Not surprisingly, there were *other* principles, which were equally as important, that didn't have anything to do with our relationship with food. Yes, it's more than just eating smart.

Make no mistake about it, my friend, a successful physical transformation—one defined by rapid and lasting change—does *not* happen haphazardly. It happens by careful design. Following a set of common principles, or the "Key Lessons" as we will so affectionately refer to them throughout the course of this book, is what separates the successful from unsuccessful transformations. From those whose body weight constantly yo-yos to those who experience satisfying and lasting weight loss. And as simple and easy as these principles might appear, I have found they're rarely used and yet surprisingly, incredibly powerful. And that is how this book came to be.

Diets Suck! begins with a chronicle based on a true story, with fictional names used for the real characters. However, throughout this book, you'll also read true transformation "success stories" of real people, with their real names and authentic photos. I thought this approach would allow you to learn more effectively by losing yourself— perhaps even *seeing yourself*—in the story and being able to better relate to the characters. It also helps to understand how these Lessons can be applied more easily, in your own "real-world" environment, where the pace of our hectic lives and daily distractions of eating unhealthy make staying on track seem impossible at times.

To help you apply the material in your own life, a brief section following the story outlines how to put everything you've learned in this book together. The final section includes a look at the most common mistakes people make when beginning a physical weight-loss transformation, and how to easily overcome them. In this section, I answer the most commonly asked questions that typically follow, after reading this book.

And thankfully, *Diets Suck!* is laid out in such a way that it won't turn your life upside down (unlike what diets do)!

Finally, it's good to keep in mind that this book is based on my work with thousands of successful clients and their families and friends, and I've found its Key Lessons are applicable for anyone interested in losing weight, transforming their bodies, and improving their health—whether 25 or 75 years old… male or female… a busy mom, truck driver, executive, or simply someone who could use some self "health" improvement.

Whatever the case may be for you, I sincerely hope it helps you transform your body, reclaim your health, and regain your life so you can achieve more than you ever imagined. That, after all, is what you deserve.

So please, let's not wait another second. **Turn the page, and let's start our journey together…**

Chapter One

AUDREY

It's 6:00 o'clock in the morning on a Saturday. The only time when the house is quiet and peaceful. Even the dogs are asleep in their kennels.

Audrey pours herself a cup of coffee, adds a generous amount of vanilla creamer, and begins to slather a blueberry bagel with a thick layer of cream cheese.

She stretches her arms out as she sits down in front of her computer. Taking a bite of her bagel, she considers the past week. Thinking about her boss, her shoulders immediately tense with frustration, and her fingers start to almost automatically type "Monster.com" in the Google search bar.

She feels her anger building up inside. *What a total jerk he was again this week*, Audrey thinks to herself. She sighs softly, as the web browser pulls up her search, and then takes a sip of her coffee. She doesn't want to dwell on last week and especially not on her boss. This is her only time, it feels like, for herself, and she doesn't want to waste it thinking about her job and that awful person!

Scrolling through the job listings in Colorado, one in particular catches her eye. "Wanted: Accountant who can keep our numbers fit!"

Intrigued, Audrey clicks the link.

Ummm… a fitness company, emerging in the nutrition field. Audrey dives in a little more, reading past the headline and job description and starts checking out the company.

Wow, she thinks to herself, the owner and founder, a man by the name of Daniel Stephens, was voted Best Boss in America. *That sounds pretty cool—the opposite of what I have now*, she mutters to herself. *Plus, the whole company looks like they're passionate about helping people… I like that*, she thinks to herself.

The list of awards they've won impresses Audrey. Entrepreneur of the Year. Outstanding Young American. Fastest Growing Company. And on and on. And the company's "leadership" management team definitely has a lot of experience in their industry.

EXTRAORDINARY CHANGES

Then Audrey notices another tab on the company's website—"Success Stories."

Curious, she clicks on the tab. After a few seconds, up comes a page where she finds "before and after" pictures of people. As she scrolls through the page, she sees there are hundreds of them. People who, by all accounts, look pretty ordinary, but who have *really* improved their bodies.

Audrey has seen "before and after" pictures like this before, and most were unbelievable to her. But, these pictures seem different. Most of them had lost a great amount of body weight. Others look like they completely resculpted their physiques. And, some had gone from looking pretty good already in their "before" pictures, in her opinion, to looking like they could now be on one of those fitness magazines she's seen at the grocery store. Still, these pictures are different from those she had seen before—splattered on the television and in magazine advertisements. These, rather, all seem *authentic* to her. They weren't celebrities, or professional athletes, or paid endorsements. They're *real* people, who had made *extraordinary* changes.

Amazing! she mutters to herself. Leaning forward in her chair, and looking closer at their "after" pictures, she exclaims out loud, "All of them look so happy and confident." Audrey starts to imagine if she could ever accomplish something like these people had.

Starting to wonder whether she'd heard the kids beginning to wake up, she quickly takes another bite of her bagel. Using her other hand to open up a desk drawer, she pulls out her résumé file. She starts reading over her cover letter. She can't believe she's doing this—that she's actually considering going through with it. She's been thinking about it for months—how much she hates her job, and boss—but hasn't had the nerve to search for another place to work, let alone follow through by submitting her résumé. She pulls up her résumé and cover letter on the computer screen, and before she has time to think about it any further, she types in the company's name on the top of the cover letter, clicks the button, "SUBMIT," and posts her cover letter and résumé to apply for the job.

With a sense of relief, she leans back in her chair, closes her eyes, and imagines what it would be like to work for a company like this…

WAKE-UP CALL

As she opens her eyes, she gazes down at her tummy and notices layers of belly fat are folding over the waistline of her sweatpants. *Gross*, Audrey mutters to herself, as she takes her fingers and grazes them across her belly. She begins to think about her weight. She weighs over 250 pounds now, after the birth of her second son. The heaviest she's ever been.

She has struggled with her weight her entire life. As long as she can remember, her weight fluctuated after trying what seems like every fad diet, magic pill, and frozen diet food, but she has never had results that lasted. She would lose a few pounds of weight, just to gain it all back, sometimes with a few *bonus* pounds.

Considering how she looks, physically, Audrey wonders if the company will take one look at her and decide she doesn't "fit" in. Her doubt is quickly overrun with excitement, as she starts thinking, dreaming… *What if I actually got the job…? Could I learn something to finally lose this ugly weight, once and for all?*

So deep in thought, she didn't even hear her husband Joe walk into the study, until his hands are on her shoulders, and he's kissing her cheek. "Good morning, honey," he whispers to Audrey. He glances at the computer screen, seeing Monster.com. "Another rough week, huh?" he asks. "Are you just dreaming, or do you think you'll apply to something this time?"

"Actually," Audrey smiles. "I just did… and the company, oh my gosh, you've got to see this…"

Chapter Two

NERVES

Stepping out of her SUV, Audrey stands to her full height of five foot ten inches. She pulls her shoulders back and tries to hold in her stomach as much as she can. She brushes her light brown hair away from her face, takes a deep breath, and walks up to the front door of the office building.

She can't believe that just one week ago, she submitted her résumé. She still feels the butterflies in her stomach from when she got the call saying they'd love to have her come in to talk about the open accounting position. Now she's just minutes away from sitting down face to face with the "Best Boss" of the company behind all those inspiring success stories. Her breath catches, and she reminds herself she *has what it takes* to get this job.

Self-consciously, she opens the front door, wondering if everyone here is going to look like "fitness models." Looking up from her desk, from behind a bouquet of colorful, exotic flowers, the office manager smiles at her warmly, introduces herself, and asks Audrey to have a seat.

Audrey notices, with a sigh of internal relief that Jocelyn, the office manager, looks healthy and vibrant, but she doesn't look like a "model." Instead, Audrey finds herself chatting with a kind, friendly, grounded woman who clearly likes to laugh. Jocelyn looks at Audrey and proclaims, "I was one of the first employees hired here. But I remember how nerve-racking it can be doing an interview. You'll do fine. Do you want something to drink, like coffee or bottled water while you wait?"

"No thanks. I'm fine. Thank you, though." Audrey feels the tension draining from her shoulders and starts to look forward to the interview, getting even more excited than when she first walked in.

THE INTERVIEW

After what seemed like an eternity, but was really only a few minutes, Audrey is invited to come into the conference room. While walking down the hallway, she notices more of the "before and after" pictures hanging on the walls, like those she had seen on the company's website. This time, though, they seem even more *real*. Maybe because the pictures have names on them and are hanging on the company's walls. *These are incredible pictures, and so inspiring*, she thinks to herself.

So taken by the photographs, Audrey almost walks by the doorway to the conference room. Abruptly, she turns and walks into a large room, well lit by the natural sunlight coming in through a wall of windows, and sits down at a large maple wood table with a shiny acrylic finish.

Moments later, the owner, Daniel Stephens—the founder and CEO of the company—walks into the room, through a connected office doorway. Strangely, Audrey feels like she already knows him, likely because she read so much about him before coming in for the interview.

Daniel is tall, with light brown, spiky hair, and is sharply dressed, wearing a black button-up polo shirt with his company's logo on the front, dark blue jeans, and a black belt with a shiny metallic buckle. He appears physically fit—sporting broad shoulders and a slim waistline. His intense smile is the first thing Audrey notices as he reaches out his hand, saying, "Welcome. Sorry for being a few minutes late, Audrey. It's very nice to meet you. I'm glad you could make it in today."

Going through the customary interview questions, and providing details on her working background, Audrey feels like the interview is going well. In fact, she hasn't stumbled on any of the questions and is confident about her knowledge in accounting.

She acknowledges the interview is coming to a close, so she figures she'd better say what's on her mind, in order to leave Daniel with a "good" impression.

"If given the opportunity," Audrey exclaims timidly yet with mild excitement, "I feel as though I could do extremely well in this position."

Then suddenly, Daniel sits up and leans toward her. "Why do you want to work here, Audrey?"

Audrey, appearing a bit caught off guard by the question, takes a deep breath, "I think I could really do a great job as your accountant…" she starts saying, but then pauses and adds, "but the most important reason I want to work here is because you genuinely seem like you want to help people. You know," her voice begins to tremble… "People like me… People who need to lose weight and improve their health and self-confidence," she says, looking down and away from Daniel.

Daniel smiles at her warmly and replies, "Thank you for being so honest. I'm glad you see that in us. Honestly, that's why we get up every morning, Audrey, and do all we do here. We're passionate about helping people build leaner, stronger, healthier bodies, so they can feel more confident and live extraordinary lives."

Standing quickly, Daniel adds, "I'd like to take you around the office, so you can meet the rest of the team. Would that be okay with you?"

Audrey nods and smiles, feeling that this is a good sign indeed.

Chapter Three

A FRESH START

A short, rushed two weeks later, Audrey pulls into the parking lot, smiling, nervous, jittery, and excited to be starting her new job. The last two weeks seem like a blur. Between the extra hours her old boss thought she *owed him* to filling out all the necessary paperwork to start her new job to running the kids to daycare and their evening activities, Audrey hadn't even had a chance to let it all sink in. Until this morning.

Waking up early, she couldn't believe how fortunate she felt. And as she hurries to get dressed and ready for her first day, the feeling comes rushing into her again. *Today is my lucky day*, she excitedly says to herself, as she pulls up in the parking spot in front of the building. Looking in the visor mirror, to check her makeup and hair, she rushes so as not to be late. Stepping out of the car, she softly mutters to herself, *I'm so ready for a fresh start!*

As Audrey tries to push down the butterflies threatening to fly out of her belly, she sees Jocelyn smiling at her as she walks into the office. She can't help but almost beam back at her as Jocelyn says, "I had hoped they would hire you! I knew you were the right choice. You're going to love it here!"

Audrey agrees wholeheartedly, laughing a bit to herself.

As she's led into a sunlit front-facing office, Audrey notices her office is right next to the conference room where she interviewed and between the chief financial officer and her new boss, Daniel. She sits down and turns on the computer sitting on the beautiful maple U-shaped desk just as Leroy, the CFO walks in, "Are you ready for all this," he drawls with a potent Texas accent and a squinting gleam in his eyes.

TIME REALLY DOES FLY

The CFO looks the part of a Texas gentleman. Finely creased blue jeans, a western-style button-up shirt, large horseshoe belt buckle, and well-shined cowboy boots cementing the impression. He starts taking her through the current projects, shows her the system and where everything resides, talks with her about what needs to be accomplished first, and introduces her more formally to the accounting staff. *Wow, I'm not going to be bored in my new job,* she thinks to herself, more than once throughout the day as she learns more about her position and the company.

Thinking it must be about lunchtime, Audrey glances at the clock and is floored to see it's after 4:00. *The day has rushed by—in a good way,* she thinks to herself. At her past job, the clock was a cruel master—as she looked at it every hour throughout the day, longing to get back to her boys, into some comfortable clothes, to settle in on the couch at home to read stories, watch movies, snack on her favorite chocolate-covered raisins, and spend time with her family.

After running some papers to her new staff, she notices Daniel's door is wide open and asks Jocelyn about this. "Oh, Daniel has an open-door policy. He's involved in just about everything here, and he likes for people to be able to ask questions when they have the need," she tells Audrey.

THE TALK

Almost reluctantly, yet filled with curiosity, Audrey pokes her head into Daniel's office and sees the back of his high black leather chair is faced away from the door, and he's focused intensely on whatever is on his computer screen. Noticing a giant plaque above Daniel's desk, written in what looks like Japanese, she wonders what it says. Afraid to interrupt him, though, she shrugs and quietly starts to turn away, just as Daniel turns his chair around, looks up, and sees her. "Audrey!" he exclaims. "Welcome to iSatori! I've been meaning to stop in to check in with you all day…to see how you're doing… We're so glad to have you here," as he smiles.

"What can I help you with?" he adds.

Not used to being treated so kindly by the owner, or anyone "above her" for that matter, Audrey is taken aback a bit by his question and feels tongue-tied. But seeing Daniel's expectant look, she blurts out, "I must ask, after seeing all the before and after photos of people you've helped transform their bodies… I hope you don't mind me asking but… *are they real*?"

It's obvious, Audrey at once wishes she could shove the sentence back into her mouth, afraid she might have just offended her new boss.

Much to her relief, Daniel just chuckles and smiles. "They do look almost unbelievable, don't they? But yes, in fact, every single one is very much real, and they each have such a unique and inspiring story to share. In fact, I can recall the story behind each transformation and the challenges they had to overcome to achieve their newfound bodies."

"What's the trick then? I mean… How did they do it?" Audrey again finds herself blurting out, without thinking first, and barely resists the urge to slap her hands over her mouth to prevent more words from rushing out unexpectedly.

"Trick?" Daniel asks rhetorically. "There's no trick, but I think you already know that," he says with a slight chuckle, as if he's answered this question a thousand times.

Instead of answering her right away, he turns slightly and stands up from this chair, and points to the plaque with the Japanese writing on the wall behind him. "The answers, however, are right there."

Chapter Four

THE "SATORI" MOMENT

"You see, our company name, iSatori, is based on the Japanese word Satori," Daniel explains as he points at the plaque. "It means to have an epiphany or an awakening. Where, once you have the answers, suddenly everything seems possible, which in our case means building a better body. We added the 'i' to make it more personal, because every transformation begins within. With you," Daniel's eyes look intently toward Audrey's.

He continues, "I believe every person, male or female, whether they're 25 or 75 years old, at some point in their life has what I call a 'Satori' moment... that's when, one day, they look in the mirror and don't like what they see—they aren't happy with their physical appearance, or how they feel, or their health... That's their awakening!

"It is this very moment, the 'Satori' moment, when people have an awakening to what *is* possible. An epiphany to what life *can* be like. And that's when it's our job to reach out a hand to help them get from where they are to where they want to be—physically and healthfully.

"And Audrey, you know what...? Each and every one of those pictures you see lined in our hallways started with that 'Satori' moment. We reached out to them, and they followed our advice... the specific advice you can see written in Japanese on the plaque hanging behind me on the wall.

"These are the '7 Lessons' to eating smart and losing weight. Permanently.

"All they had to do then was follow these Lessons for almost unbelievable weight loss," Daniel goes on, getting more and more passionate as he speaks. "And as you can clearly see, they have all changed their lives for the better as a result."

"But *how* did they do it?" Audrey quickly asks, curious.

THE HOMEWORK ASSIGNMENT

Wanting nothing more than to learn how all these people lost weight, seemingly so effortlessly, and completely transformed their bodies, Audrey, for a brief moment, finds herself shutting down. She so desperately wants to know how she could lose her own extra body weight—permanently.

Her head drops. *I don't want him to think the only reason I'm in his office is because I want to lose weight,* she thinks to herself. It's her first day on the job, and she was hired for her accounting expertise, not to learn how to lose weight herself.

Watching Audrey's body language, Daniel senses she's struggled with her weight and her self-confidence, so he turns and walks toward her, stopping a few feet away and gently says, "Audrey, while it's not 'required,' we certainly welcome and encourage everyone here to learn and to eventually live the iSatori way of life. A life filled with smart eating, exercise, and living with confidence and self-fulfillment. It's something I'm as passionate about sharing with the people I work with as with our thousands of customers."

Audrey couldn't believe what she was hearing. It was like Daniel had read her thoughts and understood her lifelong dream. *Is he really offering to help me right now?* Audrey's afraid to ask… afraid to hope after all these years of struggling.

"If you're interested, there's probably no better time than now to start learning. What do you think… are you interested?"

Audrey can hardly contain her excitement, though trying not to reveal too much emotion to Daniel.

"If so," Daniel says, stepping back, "please come on in, and have a seat." He motions with his hand to the chair in front of his desk.

Not even realizing she had been standing in the doorway for this entire conversation, Audrey moves forward and sits down in the black-cloth chair with maple wood arms. Straightening her shirt, she sits up tall and looks at Daniel expectantly. Barely able to speak, Audrey clears her throat, still afraid to appear too excited and simply nods.

"Great! That's what I was hoping," Daniel says, leaning forward, and pulling out a little black notebook from his top desk drawer, he hands it to her.

"I'd like you to do me a favor. I want you to take this book with you. Take it everywhere you go for the next three days. Each time you eat or drink something, write it down. It's important you don't try to change *anything* about the way you live or eat right now. Please, this is all so very important—I need you to be completely truthful with me and, especially, with yourself.

"This is where the journey begins. You may feel vulnerable, but you need to trust yourself and others—namely me," he smiles again. "Please don't worry. There's no judgment here. This is an important first step to your success with lifelong weight loss and vibrant health."

Again, afraid to speak, Audrey glances up and nods as she takes the black journal from Daniel. Then as she stands up and starts walking away toward the door, she turns slightly to look over her shoulder and says quietly, "Thank you."

As she walks down the hallway back toward her office, Audrey feels a tension and anxiousness in the pit of her stomach. It's a *good* feeling of positive stress, she distinguishes. It's as though she feels a sense of certainty, that "this time" is "the time" for her to lose the weight she's struggled with all her life, once and for all.

She presses the black journal against her chest, folding her arms around it, as she walks back into her office…

Chapter Five

THE NOTEBOOK

Thirty minutes later, as Audrey finishes up her work for the day, she leans back in her chair, stretching her arms over her head, and feeling a calm satisfaction for all she's accomplished during her first day.

Smiling, she picks up her purse and a few manila folders filled with documents she wants to take home to read. She laughs to herself remembering how much she dreaded "homework" from her last job. But here, she is taking stuff home on her own.

Taking a last look around her office, she sees the black book Daniel had given her earlier, sitting next to the computer keyboard. With a little anxious hesitation, she reaches for the book, places it on top of her folders, and swiftly heads out of the office for the night, eager to get back to her family and tell them how her first day went.

Driving home, Audrey thinks more about her conversation with Daniel. She can't believe he took time from his day to help her with something personal. *He doesn't even really know me yet*, she thinks to herself. She hardly even knows how to feel about it, but she tells herself she will *do her best to do everything he's asked!*

But tonight, she excitedly says to herself… *I'm going to celebrate with my family!*

DAY 1

The next morning, as Audrey finishes eating her breakfast, she takes out the black book Daniel had given her the day before and begins filling it out. She quickly writes down, "bagel with blueberry cream cheese and half of a slice of white toast with grape jelly and glass of 2% chocolate milk" (the toast and chocolate milk was actually the rest of her son Aiden's breakfast).

Getting the kids off to daycare with practiced efficiency, she heads in to the office for her next day with her Grandé mocha double-shot caramel latte with whipped cream, along with the files she read through last night, and her little black book. Just as she pulls into work, she remembers she's supposed to write down *everything* she eats *and drinks*, so she quickly writes the "latte" down before grabbing the rest of her personal belongings and running up the stairs to the office.

As she walks in, she wonders about the 7 Lessons to eating smarter and losing weight Daniel had mentioned and wishes she could read Japanese, so she could understand the writing on the plaque in Daniel's office, and she could avoid having to be lectured on how poorly she eats. Stepping into her office, she starts to feel like maybe she should eat healthier while she's filling in her black book. The thought passes, as she recalls Daniel asking her to be completely honest and not to change *any* of her eating habits.

Throughout the day, she keeps the black book with her, filling in every little thing that crosses her lips. From the two pieces of chocolate candy she took out of her purse, to the delicious, but greasy cheeseburger, fries, and tall cola she had at the nearby fast-food restaurant for lunch, to the bag of trail mix, loaded with chocolate M&M's, along with the box of crackers she keeps in her desk for snacking on in the mid-afternoon.

FEELING GRATEFUL

Barely knowing them, she already loves the ladies she works with in her department—*what fun they are to work with!* Audrey thinks to herself. They live with such passion and enthusiasm for the company and the contribution their work makes. And they know how to laugh. Her accountant has such a great sense of humor.

She can't remember the last time she smiled and even laughed out loud so much on the job—nor can she remember accomplishing so much in a single day. Everyone seems to be productive, but like they have fun while doing their work. The stress of all there is to do is certainly there, but it seems so much easier when surrounded by a pleasurable team of people who enjoy working together.

Later that evening, after dinner, clean up, bath time, and normal nightly household chores, Audrey takes a deep breath as she sits at her empty kitchen table. The kids are finally asleep, and she has some time with Joe, her husband, before she passes out in her own bed. Audrey sips on a Coke and finishes a bedtime snack—the rest of her son's macaroni and cheese from dinner, directly from the pan.

Just before wandering into the living room to sit down with her husband to watch some "grown up" television, she decides she wants something sweet, so heads out to the smaller freezer in the garage and grabs them both a root beer popsicle from her son's snacks. Remembering at the last moment, she quietly pulls out her little black book and starts writing down the remaining foods she's eaten since dinner, holding it so Joe can't easily see what she's writing.

Curious, he leans toward her anyway. "What's that?" he asks. "I don't think I've ever seen that notebook before... what are you writing?"

"Nothing... *nothing really*... I'm just doing a little homework..." Audrey feels her cheeks getting warm as she starts to blush. She's too embarrassed to tell Joe it's a food diary. He's seen her try and fail with so many diets over the years—ever since they began dating— and she doesn't want him to know she's starting what she thinks will be another "diet."

"Whatever," Joe shrugs, only semi-interested in the first place. He looks back at the TV but then laughs and retells a funny story of how Aiden, their son, had been so excited when he saw him after work, he had launched himself from the couch straight into his arms, almost knocking him over. "God, I love our boys," he tells Audrey, squeezing her shoulder briefly and leaning forward to brush his cheek against her face, again glancing at her notebook.

Audrey quickly closes the book and, as casually as possible, places it in her work bag.

Her popsicle stick rests on the coffee table in front of her, and she feels guilty already about eating it. Glancing down at her belly, she feels the usual shame. *I didn't need that,* she thinks sadly, worried about what Daniel will say when he reviews her journal. *He did ask me not to change anything yet, though, and God knows, that's how I typically eat.*

...and why you look like you do, Audrey, another voice in her head seems to add unbidden.

20

Chapter Six

THE "BLACK BOOK" REVIEW

Three days later, as Audrey sits in her car in front of the office of her new employer, she skims through the black book, and it sinks in again, how poorly she's been eating. As she glances over the items of food she wrote, she quickly realizes this type of unhealthy eating had been constant over the last several years. At least since after she and Joe had gotten married, eight years earlier.

Embarrassed, Audrey intuitively knows so much of what she eats is really bad, unhealthy foods, which she has, without a doubt, consumed to excess over the years in between the many diets she's endured. *I have no will power, and I don't know when to stop eating*, she thinks to herself as she tries to prepare herself for the lecture she just knows is coming from Daniel after he reads her black book.

Hesitantly, at the agreed upon time, she walks into Daniel's office and sits down quietly, almost hoping he won't turn around in his chair, as he finishes typing on his computer. But as if he has eyes in the back of his head, Daniel takes a deep breath and swings his chair around so he can look her in the eyes. Immediately, he reaches a hand out for the notebook, asking excitedly, "So, how'd you do?"

"What do you mean?" Audrey replies, a bit confused by his tone and his words.

Daniel laughs, "I mean, how did you do? Were you able to eat as you normally do? Were you able to write out all three days? Did you write down *everything* you ate *and* drank?"

Audrey feels the heat rising into her cheeks already as she stutters and answers quietly, "Well, yes. I mean, I did fill it out, and every single thing I ate and drank is listed. But…" Audrey hesitates. "I think…"

Anticipating her angst, before she can say anything more, Daniel interrupts, "Good. I'm glad you took this very important first step. It feels good, doesn't it?"

Confused and wondering, *where is he going with this?* Audrey blurts out, "But Daniel, it doesn't feel good at all. I ate horribly. I'm not happy about it at all. I had no idea really how poorly I've been eating." Her eyes shutting, she adds, "I'm really embarrassed…"

"Audrey," Daniel starts with a soft, compassionate tone, "there's no reason to feel embarrassed. You followed my instructions exactly. You see, I want you to understand that *no one* is perfect in how they eat. I am not. You are not. Nobody else surely is. *No one.* But I'll tell you what… the good news is, there's always room for improvement."

Looking over what she had written down, Daniel stands up from his chair and says to Audrey, excitedly, "I can see there are several small steps we can take *right away* to greatly improve how you eat. And those small steps can, in turn, make very big changes in how you look, how you feel, and in your health. Would you like that?"

Audrey nods, still looking down and still feeling a bit ashamed.

SURRENDER

"First, before we start on our journey together," Daniel then interrupts himself, "you do understand this is a journey, right?" looking at Audrey for acknowledgment, seeing her nod slightly, he continues. "You realize there is no *silver bullet* for losing weight. There is no magic pill that does all the work for you. You won't find your new body in a frozen meal plan or inside a secret book or on an online forum… You've already tried all those things in the past, haven't you?" he asks almost rhetorically as if he's made this "speech" before. "Those things haven't worked out so well, have they? Look what they've brought you… a life of yo-yo dieting, watching your weight go up and down and back up and probably feeling hopeless…" Audrey can only nod her head in agreement, her eyes sad and distant, as she remembers all her failed attempts.

"Audrey," Daniel exclaims, startling Audrey with his increased volume from the soft words of a second before. "Tell me some of the words that reflect how you've felt about yourself and the constant yo-yo dieting you've put yourself through over the years?"

Hesitating for just a breath, thinking to herself, *This is hard, but you can do it, Audrey. Don't cry. Dad taught you not to show weakness, especially in front of your new boss.*

Pulling her chin up, as casually as possible so Daniel doesn't notice, Audrey wipes under her eyes with her fingers, ensuring no tears are falling or leaving telltale black streaks of mascara. She musters up all the courage she has to tell Daniel exactly how she's felt all the years she's been dieting, so unsuccessfully.

"It's been a constant struggle.

"I've felt frustrated.

"Depressed.

"Sad.

"Unaccepted.

"And I definitely lack confidence in myself."

Hesitating, Daniel can see her internal struggle in her eyes. "Is there more?" Daniel asks gently but with genuine curiosity.

"No. Not really. I mean. I don't think so… Yeah, that's it." Audrey finally decides.

Glancing out the window and then allowing his gaze to return to Audrey's face, Daniel says, "Really? I sense there might be something more you'd like to share… maybe to just get it off your chest?"

AUDREY'S SATORI MOMENT

Audrey can't hold it back any longer, and she feels the small tears starting to roll down her cheeks. But to her complete surprise, she realizes she doesn't feel uncomfortable at all. Instead, she's relieved to finally be able to get it all off her chest.

Leaning forward, almost like she's about to whisper a secret, she begins quietly, reluctantly, "I feel… I feel…" she starts to stutter and then sniffles, "I feel... as though my husband wishes I weren't so fat. I don't think he finds me... attractive, I guess, though he's afraid to say it... because he doesn't want to hurt my feelings."

Stunned, Daniel leans back. He's been through this exercise with many, many people over the years, but never has someone been so authentic and so vulnerable. Realizing with great gratitude and humility, he's witnessing Audrey's "Satori moment," right here in his office.

This is *it* for her. Her moment. *The* moment that will change her life forever, from this point forward...

Chapter Seven

THE RELEASE

Daniel feels a mixture of enthusiasm and sadness. Looking at Audrey, he's filled with excitement, knowing she's finally surrendered to her feelings of how being overweight has held her back in so many areas of her life and how she's now ready to accept a new life. One free of the burden of being overweight and the feelings of inadequacy that have come hand in hand with the weight and how she sees herself and her body.

On the other hand, Daniel feels the sense of sadness he experiences every time he thinks about the hundreds of thousands of men and women who, just like Audrey, feel the same way she does about their weight and themselves. But who have not yet gotten to this important point in their lives, where they're ready to surrender to their feelings.

Admiringly, Daniel is astonished that Audrey, a brand new employee, has made herself so vulnerable. He's proud she's taken this life-changing step and can't hold back to tell her.

Politely, yet sternly, he says, "Audrey, I've been helping people—lots and lots of people—for many, many years change their bodies. I want you to know that what you just did... sharing your vulnerability... your authenticity… your ability to pull out those deep-rooted feelings—was a magical moment. I hope you recognize that. I'm very proud of you." Daniel feels his eyes shine with enthusiasm.

Looking back at him, as she wipes the remaining tears from underneath her eyes and off her cheeks, she smiles back. Her eyes say thank you, without her having to utter a word.

"Audrey, I want you to remember this moment. Okay?" Daniel asks. "This is the first, most important step to changing the way you look at yourself… you surrendered to your feelings… I'm really in awe of you right now and the fantastic journey I *know* you're now beginning.

"This is the first and most important step to changing your appearance—how you look and how you feel. You'll always look back at this moment as the defining moment in your life, and I'm so grateful to have shared it with you. It's exciting. Now, you'll have to agree with me this time, I think," Daniel adds smiling, "It feels *good*, doesn't it?"

Audrey, looking *and feeling* as though she had just unloaded a thousand-pound weight off her shoulders, sighs and says, "Daniel, oh my goodness, yes. It's such a relief to have finally gotten all of that off my chest. Honestly, I don't think I even knew myself how I felt. It's like I've been burying all those feelings and emotions deep down inside, beneath this layer of body fat. Afraid to acknowledge it even existed. Now I don't know why I didn't think I could face it. I feel… like I'm lighter. Freer. Like I can do something now to finally change…

"I've felt pent up for *so, so long.* So many years. But I didn't have any way to release it." Laughing, Audrey adds, "I feel like I'm ready to sprint around the building. I have so much ENERGY!"

Looking directly at Daniel, she says, "Thank you. Daniel, thank you so very much." And leaning forward even more, she exclaims, with greater confidence in her body and voice than he's witnessed since he met her, and likely more than she's shown in years, "This is it. I can feel it. I can do it NOW! I know I can!"

"Is it too much to ask for the next step?" Audrey blurts out.

Daniel, with an even bigger answering smile, replies, "You are ready, Audrey. You are! Let's start our journey together. But first, there's just one more thing I need to ask you, and I need an absolutely honest answer from you…"

Chapter Eight
THE COMMITMENT

Though he looks like he can't hold back another smile, Daniel refrains and looks serious. Audrey's body language and demeanor immediately mirrors his, and while she still feels that lightness, she is instantly washed over with a sense of calm.

"Audrey," Daniel begins, with almost doctor-like authority, "I need to ask you a very serious question…

"Are you *committed* to making this change?"

Sitting back in his high-backed black chair, looking directly at her, he adds, "I mean, are you *really, truly, honestly committed*, Audrey? 100%… Are you willing to give this everything you've got?"

"Because while I can share what I've learned to help you, you will be doing all the 'work' yourself. You'll do the 'heavy lifting,' pardon the pun, but will also reap all the rewards."

Daniel goes on, "Will you listen to the advice I have to share? Will you be honest with me, and even more importantly, will you be honest with yourself—even when you slip up? Because you *will* slip up. We all slip up."

He looks at Audrey expectantly, eagerly awaiting her response. "I need to know you're *fully* committed to taking the steps necessary to achieve the body and health you've always dreamed you could have. So again, are you committed fully?" Daniel asks, reading Audrey's body language as he listens for her response.

Motionless, Audrey is no longer fidgeting as she was just moments before. Daniel still feels her mild sense of anxiety, but senses it's starting to calm now.

"Daniel…" she says, her voice steady, but then she pauses and looks up as if considering her words carefully. "Daniel, I'm in. 100%!"

Distracted by her own internal musings, she can hardly put the words together. "I've waited…" She starts over, nervous to get the answer out… "I've waited almost my entire adult life. For this… moment." Her speech catching up to her words, she adds, as she clears her throat, "I can't remember the last time I felt this eager to start anything new in my life. Well…" she says smiling, "Except for this job…

"You have my word. I will commit myself entirely to our journey together. I know, Daniel, I will reach my goal of losing this ugly weight I've been carrying around all of my life… of feeling lighter, more energetic, becoming healthier, and … and of finally being happy with the reflection I see in the mirror."

Clearly, in that moment, Audrey had achieved a renewed sense of hope. Her new enlightenment was guiding her thoughts.

"Good. Because if I sensed in the least, Audrey, that this was just a momentary excitement and you weren't fully committed, then we wouldn't be able to go any further than where we are today. I can tell, though, you are committed to this lifestyle change. *Very* committed," Daniel shares.

Standing from his chair, Daniel places his hand on his own chest and opens his mouth to ask what is clearly another important question…

Chapter Nine
LOVE THYSELF

"Audrey, what do you think of yourself?" he begins.

"Do you *love* yourself?" his eyes gaze intently into Audrey's, as if he's reaching for something deeper in her.

Relaxing slightly, he steps back, "This isn't part of my program, but I think it's an important question for each of us to ask ourselves from time to time."

Unsure of his motive now, Audrey feels the excitement start to drain. Looking away, somewhat embarrassed, she answers, "I don't." Her lips frown. "I'm sorry. But no, I don't think I love myself."

Walking away from his chair, almost as if he didn't hear what she said, he walks around his desk until he's directly in front of Audrey. Then leans back against his desk, just a couple of feet in front of her, and goes on to ask, "Do you have any photographs of yourself? Like in your purse or at your desk? Just one picture. It can be of just you or of you with your family. It doesn't matter—as long as it's current."

Still puzzled by his last question, and Daniel's new request, she has to think for a moment before she blurts, "Yes. I do!" She reaches into her small leather purse, "Wait a second," she says, pulling out her wallet and flipping it open to reveal a picture of her sitting with her two sons, smiling brightly as they're laughing. Daniel smiles as he sees the joy on their faces.

"Here you go," Audrey says as she hands Daniel the photo.

Daniel pulls his hand back, saying, "No… I want you to keep it. But there's something very important I'd like you to do with it. Please take this picture and hang it up in your office. Someplace where you'll be able to clearly see it throughout the day. Like taped to your computer monitor or right next to your phone on your desk."

Clinching the photo between her fingers, Audrey smiles too, loving the looks on her children's faces. But then she begins to frown, as she notices in the photo how her belly bunches up at her waist and how she looks so *frumpy* and *flabby* in her mind.

Looking up, she asks, "But then, won't other people see it too?"

THE POWER OF A PICTURE

"That's okay," Daniel answers. "That's part of the program. You may not believe me now, but when we're done, you'll actually be very proud of that picture, and you may even want more people to see it. Trust me on that," his eyes sparkle knowingly.

Thoroughly perplexed now, Audrey looks up at Daniel curiously, but doesn't know how to tell him she's not comfortable putting the picture out for just anyone to see.

"So Audrey, here's what I would like you to do with that photo,"

Daniel explains. "Three times a day, *every single day*—maybe once in the morning, once at around lunchtime, actually, right before you leave to eat lunch… it's really important that you look at it right before you leave for lunch… and finally before you go home for the night. Do you think you can do that?"

Audrey nods.

"Now, whenever you look at this photo, I want you to say to yourself—either in your head, or better yet, out loud so it's even more powerful, '*I love my family. I love myself. I love my body.*'"

"Do you think you can do that… every day… for me, for you?" Daniel asks empathetically.

Nodding again, Audrey indicates she can do it. But Daniel also sees the perplexed look on her face about this advice.

Convincingly, Daniel leans in toward Audrey and softly says to her, "It's important for you to remember today as your Satori moment. *Never* forget what you feel like. Because today is the first day of your *new* life."

The volume of his voice increasing with his excitement, Daniel adds, "Well then, it's time to get started. Let's begin our journey together…

"And recall, there are seven Lessons in all. So why don't we meet each week, where I'll share a new Lesson, on creating a life-changing weight-loss transformation."

Turning back toward his computer, Daniel opens Outlook on his screen and searches his schedule. "How do Monday afternoons at 5 o'clock work for you, after the end of our day? Can you come into my office every week around this time? It should take no more than 30 minutes together, and we can discuss one Lesson each week.

"Each time we meet, you'll learn *exactly* how you can put each one into practice quickly to lose unhealthy weight and begin to change the way you look at yourself and the way the world sees you… one week at a time. Sound good?"

Barely able to contain her excitement, pulling her iPhone out of her purse, Audrey opens up her schedule and quickly replies that time works for her. "Can you send a meeting invite? Oh, you already did…" Clicking the button to accept the meeting, Audrey returns her phone to her purse.

"Well, this has been a pretty amazing meeting, and a great start to your transformation, wouldn't you agree?" Daniel asks.

"It's not what I expected," Audrey admits. "I thought I'd be listening to an hour of being lectured on my eating habits and how I'll never reach my goals with my current diet…" her voice trails off.

"Yeah, well, I don't think that would have been a good use of my time *or yours*. You did what you needed to do. We both know where you're starting from. That's important. And I'm excited to start seeing the changes in the upcoming weeks.

"I must admit, although some of these changes might seem incredibly simple, let's make no mistake, they are profoundly powerful once applied."

Audrey looks up at Daniel expectantly, "How soon will I see any changes… I mean…"

Nodding, Daniel says, "Now that you're committed to making the changes, I think you'll be surprised how quickly you will see results."

Looking at the clock abruptly, Daniel says, "Sorry, Audrey. I've got an important call I can't miss." Smiling, he adds. "Monday… we'll really dig in to the first Lesson. Don't forget to hang up your photo and repeat that phrase. Every day. Got it?"

"Got it," Audrey says as she gathers her purse and the photo, thrilled by the conversation she's just had with Daniel.

Her entire drive home, filled with anticipation, Audrey can't stop wondering what the next week will bring…

THE LESSONS

Chapter Ten

WEEK ONE

Monday afternoon, the sun is quickly setting over the horizon as Audrey gazes out the conference room windows. It's been sunny all day, but as it's early Spring, there's still a chill in the air, and Audrey wraps her sweater around her shoulders more tightly as she watches the wind pick up outside. As the day is coming to a close, Audrey glances anxiously toward Daniel's closed door, hearing muffled voices as he concludes a conference call.

Audrey doesn't really mind staying late today, or any day for that matter, at her new company. But today she's especially excited because she'll be learning the first, of seven, Lesson from Daniel.

As she waits for Daniel to finish up, Audrey decides to get up and walk down the hallway outside his office, looking again at the remarkable, almost unbelievable "before" and "after" transformation pictures hanging on the walls. She's drawn to one set of pictures in particular. A man by the name of Albert Rivera. She stares intensely at his images. Amazingly, Albert had lost over 100 pounds and now looks *completely* different. It's as if the "after" picture is of a completely different person than the "before" picture—that's how much Albert has transformed the way his body looks.

"Wow," she softly says to herself. "I wonder if *I* could do that?"

"Without a doubt!" exclaims Daniel, startling Audrey, as he walks up from behind.

"*Really*... You think I can?" she asks, hoping she doesn't sound desperate.

"*Absolutely*! If he can do it, so you can you, Audrey," he answers quickly. With an expression of complete certainty on his face, he adds, "You are capable of so much more than you think. In fact, today we are going to help you discover that you are actually *closer* than you might believe to achieving a spectacular weight-loss transformation like Albert did."

Audrey stands perplexed, wondering why Daniel thinks she's "close" to her weight-loss desires. "What do you mean...? I'm not sure I understand... I'm closer than I think?" she quizzes.

"Let me explain. Let's go back into the conference room and sit down. But before we do, would you do me a favor and take Albert's picture off the wall and bring it with you please?" Daniel asks.

Audrey obliges, taking the picture carefully off the wall, and follows Daniel back into the conference room. As she begins to sit down, Daniel doesn't hesitate and starts talking, "I know you can experience something similar to, heck, *even better*, than what Albert did. I know this, Audrey, because I've witnessed it firsthand with thousands of other people already.

"Let's talk about what made Albert's transformation so successful," Daniel begins as he leans back casually in his chair.

"Eating smart was important and so was regular exercise, but those weren't the most important factors to Albert's success. It was something *much deeper* and internal for him. Let me share his incredible story with you, first, so we can put everything into context…"

ALBERT THE GREAT

Speaking almost like a newscaster, Daniel begins, "Albert Rivera grew up in the Bronx, New York, where he lived like a king. Not the kings and queens you and I think about back in medieval days. He grew up with a big family. Brothers, sisters, aunts, uncles, grandparents. There wasn't a day he could remember not having his family around him while growing up. And with that big family came big gatherings and 'family-style' feasts. Every night for dinner, they would gather and have a table full of food. Huge plates piled with pasta, rice, potatoes, and lots and lots of meat, mainly beef. For Albert, and the rest of the family, eating only 'one serving' was frowned upon. It was normal to eat three or four servings at one sitting, which might last two or three hours, as they socialized and enjoyed being together.

"By the age of 24, while in his third year of college, Albert had ballooned up to 254 pounds. Keep in mind, he is only five foot seven. His waist expanded beyond a size 40, about the time when he stopped counting, or caring really. In speaking with Albert, he once said to me, *'At this weight, I hated to be part of pictures and started losing my self-confidence, due to my excessive weight. I was slipping into a reclusive, almost depressive state.'*

"But that wasn't it for him—it got even worse," Daniel continued with Albert's story.

"His doctor told him he was developing high blood pressure and would eventually need to start taking medication if he continued to gain weight. He developed sleep apnea. And worse, he was starting to develop early signs of arthritis."

"But he's only in his twenties!" Audrey blurts out, genuinely surprised.

"True," Daniel replies. "All of these awful conditions, brought on by his excessive eating and unhealthy body weight, at only 24 years old!"

Continuing to share Albert's story, Daniel went on, "What was really sad is that Albert is an accomplished jazz musician—a saxophone artist—and he loves to practice and play live concerts more than anything else in life. But his frequent bouts of arthritis made his hands hurt so badly he had a hard time playing his instrument. Sadly, he didn't know what to do about his rising weight, let alone his arthritis, and he actually told me he thought it would just 'go away over time.' Sadly, it only got worse as his weight increased.

"It wasn't long before, rather than fighting it, Albert started to think this was just the way it—that is, life and his health—were meant to be as he started aging past adolescence. He began to basically 'accept it' and figured he would simply adjust to it and 'live with it.'"

Turning ever so slightly in his chair as he switches the direction his legs are crossed, Daniel gazes out the glass wall of windows. Audrey has noticed he stares in this direction whenever he's starting to get emotional. Clearing his throat, Daniel continues, "Albert was becoming depressed. He desperately wanted to change and knew he needed to save his own life, but no matter how hard he tried to get started making positive changes, he couldn't find the type of encouragement or support he needed from his family to continue. This was very difficult for Albert. He couldn't understand why his family would always pull him back into his past, unhealthy ways of living and eating every time he tried to move forward in a positive direction.

"When we spoke about his family, Albert told me, '*It's as if they didn't want me to succeed... to live a healthier lifestyle... to lose weight. I think they felt as if they'd lose me or like I was trying to become better than them by not accepting our family's traditional ways of eating and living, when in fact all I was trying to do was to better myself... to make some positive lifestyle changes that would help me lose a few pounds and hopefully make my arthritis go away, so I could play my saxophone free of any pain. That's all I wanted, but my family just couldn't find it in their hearts to support me. It was like I alienated them. And so, sadly, without their support or approval, I fell back into my unhealthy ways of living, so they would accept me again.*'"

Turning directly to look at Audrey, Daniel asks almost rhetorically, "Can you see, Audrey, how having support is so *vitally* important to your success in losing weight, especially the support of your closest family members? That is your first Lesson."

Getting up from his chair, Daniel points to the first line on the Japanese plaque on his wall in his office. "Lesson Number One," Daniel says, "the first and most important Lesson of the seven."

Then Daniel walks briskly over to the glass white board on the wall near the front of the conference room, where he grabs a blue marker. He proceeds to write on the board:

LESSON #1: FIND A SUPPORT SYSTEM

You must find truly caring and compassionate support to help encourage and reinforce your positive lifestyle changes.

Audrey reads what he's written on the board and scurries to write it down in her own little black book.

Daniel underlines the word support, as he looks over at Audrey, and says, "Support. It's a key part of making any positive changes in your life, including losing weight and avoiding the dieting trap, and becoming healthier. It helps encourage and reinforce your positive lifestyle changes. I can't understate its importance, though it might sound incredibly simple."

A FAMILY OF FRIENDS

Daniel returns to the conference table and sits back down in his chair, as he continues to share Albert's story, "Thankfully, Albert found the support he needed, *from friends.* See, Albert lived in New York City, where he had access to a pretty robust downtown, as you can imagine, and it was there he found his 'support system'—through his *closest* friends. They knew how depressed he was becoming about his weight and the pain of not being able to play his saxophone. They encouraged him to start working out and would accompany him to the gym, to play pick-up basketball games. And they encouraged him to start taking walks through downtown as a simple way of exercising.

"The challenge for Albert was that even though he found support through his friends, he still didn't find acceptance from his family. But instead of using this as a reason *not* to change, he decided, this time, to use it as a reason *to* change his lifestyle."

Daniel went on with a look of sincerity and seriousness on his face, "But you know, Audrey, it wasn't until Albert had his 'Satori' moment that he decided to make his change permanent. Albert recounted the day with crystal clarity, as if it were yesterday when he shared the story with me…

'It was March 14, 2011, and a new fitness center was opening up at the end of my block, and I decided to join on their grand opening day. I woke up that morning, and after taking a shower, I looked in the mirror and saw myself with a renewed sense of excitement. Something inside told me this time it was going to happen. This time I was going to succeed. I felt every previous excuse I used had run its course. I felt if I didn't change this day, I would never change. I walked into the gym and said to myself it was time to start living. I was done surviving the old way. And knowing I had a strong support system of friends to encourage and motivate me along the way, I knew I was going to be a new man from that moment on.'

Picking up Albert's inspiring before and after photos off the table and turning them around so Audrey could see them, Daniel continues, "When Albert started working out, and eating smarter, his goals were simple: Make it four weeks without quitting. Lose a couple of pounds, lower his blood pressure, and he was hopeful he could reduce the stiffness in his hands so he could play his saxophone without pain."

Sitting firmly up in his chair, almost like a proud father talking about his kids, Daniel announces to Audrey, "Seven months, and what seemed like a brief moment in time later, Albert found himself weighing a much lighter and healthier 160 pounds."

Seeing the surprise on Audrey's face, Daniel reaffirms, "Yes, he had lost over 100 pounds. His waist size went down 10 sizes, to a slim 30. Just as important, his blood pressure went back to normal, healthy ranges; and to his amazement, his arthritis, which once made him feel useless as a musician, became a distant memory."

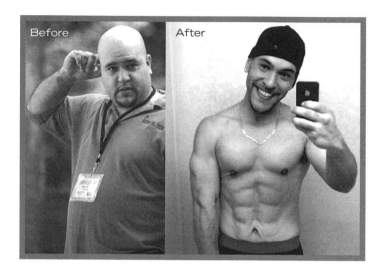

"Even more extraordinarily," Daniel goes on, even more excited than before, "Albert found his most meaningful support group of all… *his family*. They became so impressed with the changes he made in his physical appearance and his attitude about life. After only a few months, they slowly and though somewhat hesitantly at first, eventually became the biggest believers in Albert. They began to support his new way of life, encouraging him along the way by serving healthier foods when he came over for dinner. They started encouraging him to go to the gym on days he didn't feel motivated. His family *finally* turned their attention to the positive changes Albert was making and showed their deep love for him by caring for and supporting him during his transformation."

You know what's even more amazing, Audrey?" Daniel asks, not waiting for a reply, "Seven months after Albert began his life-changing experience, he entered and completed an Urbanathalon, which is a nine and half mile run through the inner city. Two years later, he crossed the finish line of his first 26.2-mile marathon… a full marathon… something he would have never imagined doing just a few months earlier."

"Best of all, Audrey," Daniel went on, getting more and more energized as he spoke, "Today, Albert is eating healthy, each and every day; touring the United States playing jazz concerts; and in his spare time, enjoying being one of our most popular 'success coaches' on our Facebook page [at www.Facebook.com/iSatoriTech], where he provides encouragement and support for those seeking help while they make their own transformations. He even started his own online social community on Facebook, called Journey2Transform, where he supports other people who need support or motivation to transform their physical health, like he did.

"When I recently spoke with Albert, he told me this about his new life, and before we ended our call, he said…

'I wake up smiling every day. I love being one of iSatori's success stories where people see me, and it gives them a feeling of hope… of what dedication and focus can bring you with the right direction. My support system continues to grow, as I continue my new way of life and expand my friendships online and at iSatori's Facebook page. I've changed my life for the better. It's a permanent lifestyle change. I'm never, ever, ever going back. And now it's time for me to pay it forward and help others walk in my footsteps. Because, if I can do it, so can they.'

As Daniel peers over at Audrey, he notices she's intently gazing at Albert's before and after pictures. After a few moments of silence, she looks up at Daniel, and proclaims, "I understand… I understand the importance of having a strong foundation… a support system. Having people who support you…who encourage you… who truly care about you… It's key to getting started and getting through the tough days along the transformation journey."

"So, Audrey, I'm glad you have grasped this first and very important Lesson. Now, are you ready for your homework?"

Audrey sighs to herself, thinking… *Geez, I thought I was done with this homework stuff.* But nods anyway.

THE HOMEWORK ASSIGNMENT

Daniel proceeds with instructions for this homework assignment, "Tonight, I want you to go home and sit your family down at the kitchen table, and tell them you really need their support. Tell them you are getting ready to start a journey, which will entail a new way of living, a new way of eating that is going to make you healthier, happier, help you lose weight, and give you lots more energy… and you are going to count on them for encouragement and their support during this lifestyle transformation. Tell them it's really important they not judge you, but simply support you unconditionally. Make sure they all agree they can help support you. Can you do this tonight?" Daniel asks as if he can't accept anything other than a yes.

"Yes… Yes, I can. I will, tonight," Audrey replies. Looking at her watch, Audrey exclaims, "I have to run now. It's time to pick up my boys—if I'm after 6:30… well, you know how it is." Pausing, she looks at Daniel, "I'll ask my family for their support, tonight at dinner… " as she smiles and then packs up her bag to rush out the door.

But just before she leaves, she turns back to look at Daniel… "Next Monday… same time? I can't wait to learn the next Lesson."

Daniel smiles and nods in agreement.

As she drives home, Audrey starts to feel a little anxious, wondering how the conversation with her family will turn out. She begins to rehearse what she's going to say to them. She stops, momentarily, to think about how great it is that she's now learning these valuable, life-changing Lessons. As curiosity begins to settle in, she starts to speculate about what the second Lesson might be…

Chapter Eleven
WEEK TWO

As she walks into the conference room the following Monday, Audrey thinks back over the past week. As she had promised Daniel, she had sat down with her family and told them about her new journey to lose weight and told them it was to "transform the way Mommy looks and feels" and asked them for their support and encouragement.

When she did it, she was hesitant, afraid her husband Joe would just roll his eyes, disbelievingly thinking, *here she goes again… another diet; start today, done tomorrow.* Instead, he did something different that completely stunned Audrey—he had reached across the table and took her hand in his. Remembering his words as if he were stating them now, she can only smile…

"Audrey, you're the most beautiful woman I know—and I love you just the way you are. But if you want to do this, then I'll… we'll… support you every step of the way." Then he leaned back and chuckled, as he rubbed his own belly, and suggested he might just benefit a little too by joining her.

Knowing she could use the support wherever she could get it, Audrey also met with her mom and sister for lunch over the weekend and asked them for their support. Like with Joe and the kids, she had hoped they would be supportive, but she didn't really expect it. They both had seen her try and fail at so many diets in the past, but again, just by asking and being vulnerable and authentic in her request for support, she found they were more than willing to be there for her and provide love and encouragement however they could. And, they even asked a lot of questions about what she was doing, because she seemed so darn excited.

What's more, they were interested to learn from Audrey that it was her new boss, the CEO and owner of the health and fitness company, who was taking the time to personally help her learn what she needed to do to transform her body.

VIRTUAL SUPPORT

Though a bit hesitant to join in their conversations, Audrey also found a much larger support system—a group of over 40,000 other people (and growing daily), on the company's online community at Facebook.com/iSatoriTech.

Once signed up, she was immediately greeted with open arms and connected with a "success coach" from her own company, iSatori. She knew who it was but acted like she didn't, nor did she give away that she was a new employee there, because she didn't want any "special" treatment.

She was astonished at the number of people who, like her, were there for support, encouragement, and friendly accountability from the lively community of members. Audrey certainly didn't feel alone.

This was encouraging. She also discovered they did more than this. In fact, the "success coaches" at iSatori provided a number of members with advice on a range of topics—from food choices to workouts to emotional support to supplements and more—giving them straightforward, no-nonsense answers. She liked that and knew she would be counting on them for lots of help. The community immediately felt like her "virtual family."

Another nice surprise for Audrey, she also buddied up with Jocelyn, the office manager, as her new "workout partner." She had watched Jocelyn heading out every day at lunch, religiously, for her workouts. Though nervous, Audrey built up the courage to ask if she could tag along. Jocelyn seemed happy to have a new partner, and during the past week, Audrey had learned how much fun it was to work out with a friend. Ironically, she now looked forward to their lunchtime activities more than she had ever looked forward to going out to eat.

GETTING EVEN BETTER

Sitting down in the conference room, Audrey feels comfortable knowing she has four strong and deeply caring support systems ready to help her along this new journey. Looking up, she notices it's 5:00 on the nose, just as Daniel comes striding out of his office, holding a folder in his hands.

Smiling, Daniel asks how the week went, and Audrey shares how supportive her family has been and that she even found additional support from others around her. Daniel then comments on how fresh and awake Audrey's eyes are and how clear her skin is and then adds, "I've seen you heading out with Jocelyn at lunchtime. So… it looks like you might have found some support around here too," he says knowingly.

"Yes!" Audrey exclaims. "I never would have thought I would enjoy working out, but Jocelyn and I have had so much fun. And you know, it's a great way to release stress during the middle of a hectic day!"

Daniel chuckles as he replies, "Yes. I definitely know that! Personally, I wake up at 5:15 a.m. every morning and work out first thing in the morning. I find it wakes me up, gets my blood flowing, my muscles moving, and my body and brain feeling alive. By the time I get to the office, I'm alert and ready to take on the day."

Setting the folder down on the table in front of him, Daniel sits slowly, saying, "My legs are still a bit sore from Friday's workout." Looking at Audrey. "As you mentioned, working out is a terrific way to relieve the stress of a hectic week, especially one like last week!

"In fact," Daniel extends the thought, "There are plenty of credible scientific studies that prove moderate exercise is a terrific way to relieve stress, reduce anxiety, help you enjoy a more restful night's sleep, and even relieve depression."

Audrey smiles as she realizes another benefit she hadn't thought of. "Interestingly, in only the last week I've been working out with Jocelyn, I've already noticed I feel better, have more energy, less stress, and although I hadn't thought about it, I *am* getting a better night's sleep lately too!"

Picking up the file on the conference table, Daniel remarks, "You know, speaking of stress, Jocelyn has quite a remarkable story too. Has she shared any of it with you?"

Surprised, Audrey responds, "No. I mean, she said she just started working out seriously about a year ago, but I don't know her story at all."

"Well, I double checked with her earlier today, and she told me I could share her story… if it might help someone else. So I get to do the honors…" Daniel says as he opens the folder he had brought in, and pulls out two pictures. One of the Jocelyn Audrey recognizes, and another picture where she looks much different.

STRESSED AND SCARED

"Has Jocelyn told you much about her family?" seeing Audrey shake her head side to side, Daniel continues.

"Well, a few years ago, Jocelyn had a scare in the middle of the workday here. She had to immediately rush out of the office after she was called and told her husband was being taken to the hospital. We weren't sure what was going to happen. But from all indications, it didn't look good. I can tell you, it was a scary and stressful time."

"I can't imagine how Jocelyn must have felt," Audrey blurts out. Daniel shakes his head, in agreement.

"That day, Rodger, her husband, had a serious stroke," Daniel says, followed by a long pause. "Fortunately, he did recover. But the stroke left him almost… I guess the best way to describe it is, almost childlike. Rodger can no longer work or fully take care of himself."

Daniel pauses again and turns to look outside.

"So on top of all the stress we pile on Jocelyn here at the office, it was much more stressful for her at home now as well.

"Jocelyn has always been a hard worker, so like most of us, she was really busy and worked a lot of extra hours. The added stress and time required of her for work and taking care of her husband, whom she loved so dearly, became almost unbearable. And because of that, she stopped taking care of herself. She stopped going on her daily walks.

She stopped eating fresh food, and she became dependent on processed, packaged, convenience foods. She never felt like she had time to go visit her granddaughters, whom she was so close to prior to Rodger's life-changing stroke.

"As the stress of her husband's illness and recovery built up, she also found her weight increasing. So much so, her weight was now approaching 200 pounds, at only five foot three inches, and her size 18 clothes were getting, as she told me... *so tight, and very uncomfortable, I didn't even want to leave my house some mornings.*"

Audrey shifts uncomfortably in her seat, and Daniel realizes how much she's relating to Jocelyn's story.

"On top of that, Jocelyn felt like she had hardly any energy, and she was becoming more and more aggravated by the simplest of things, and experiencing on and off feelings of depression.

"While her health wasn't suffering yet, after watching her husband fight to recover, Jocelyn soon realized if *she* didn't change her ways, she might not be there to give *him*, her husband, the help he so desperately needed. She was, after all, his number-one caregiver, and he depended on her almost completely."

Reading from what looks like a small essay in the folder, Daniel quotes something Jocelyn had written for him...

'*I felt awful. I knew I looked bad. I hated seeing myself that heavy. And I knew if I didn't do something soon, I wouldn't be around to take care of Rodger. I couldn't stand having this thought. I knew it was time to do something, but what... what do I do... how do I do it... I felt stuck...*'"

Audrey, looking shocked, covers her mouth and remarks, "I had no idea! I thought she had always been... well, so energetic, vibrant, and full of life. Just like she is now. I mean, she looks so amazing now. Heck, I can't even keep up with her when we work out together."

Audrey continues, "She's mentioned she has her challenges at home with her husband, but I never knew the extent."

Daniel looks back at Audrey with a serious expression and says, "I know, huh? She *is* amazing and has certainly turned things around in her life. It's hard for even me to believe this is the same woman, and I've worked with her daily for over 12 years now."

Audrey replies, "I can't even imagine her feeling depressed. I mean, stressed… aren't we all with as busy as it is around here? But Jocelyn's so… well… so together. She's virtually always willing to help anyone out, and she does it with a smile and often a laugh. And even when she's rushing through the halls, she seems energetic and confident. So… purposeful. I just can't imagine her any other way!"

"Do you know why, Audrey?

"Do you know what Lesson Jocelyn's story is here to teach us?" Daniel asks intently.

JOCELYN'S LESSON

"Ummm… I think it's because she needed to get healthy. I mean, she had to, right? She needed to, so she could be around for her husband, to take care of him," Audrey rebuts.

"Close, Audrey! The Lesson here for us is that Jocelyn didn't *need* to change, she *wanted* to change. More than anything else. And she did so, because she found her deep-rooted 'why.' And it's the 'why' that's a *very* important part of any transformation. You see, you have to unlock your reasons for wanting to change. Without your why, your deeply strong reasons, you don't have the guidance to pull you in the direction of your goals.

"As Jocelyn once confided to me," Daniel read again from the paper he was reading, written by Jocelyn…

'I really wanted to start feeling better. To get my stress and depression under control without having to resort to harmful, addictive prescription drugs; or worse, to give up altogether and have to put my husband in a full-time caretaker's home. I knew if I started exercising and feeding my body smarter, I would start feeling better and become healthier and more energetic. And because I'm the primary caretaker for my husband, I knew I had to get into better physical shape and improve his eating habits as well if we were going to live a long, fruitful life together.'"

Daniel stands up and walks over to the plaque, hanging on the wall. Audrey still can't figure out why he points to this board, because everything is written in Japanese, and she has no clue what it says.

Nevertheless, Daniel points to what appears to be the second line of words and says to Audrey, "Lesson Number Two… here it is," Daniel says as he squeezes his hand into a fist in front of his chest. "It's the one that will grip your heart, every time."

Daniel then walks over to the nearby white board, grabs a marker, and proceeds to write down the next lesson, right below the first he wrote last week…

LESSON #2: KNOW YOUR WHY

Unlock your reasons, and know your why, to draw you toward your transformation goals.

Tilting her head, Audrey looks searchingly into Daniel's face. "Okay, so she found her reason, but *what* did she do then? I mean, she must have lost, what... 50 pounds?" she says, pointing at Jocelyn's pictures.

"You're getting pretty good at this, Audrey," Daniel answers with a broad smile. "You hit it exactly. Jocelyn dropped 50 pounds of unhealthy body weight and now wears a very comfortable size 10.

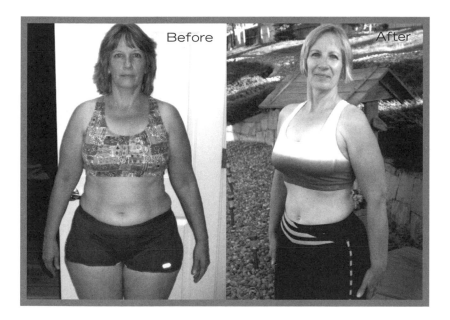

"At nearly 58 years young, she's finally comfortable with her body. She likes her weight, likes the way her clothes fit her, and loves the energy she has. I think she would tell you, though, that she still has to fight off a lot of stress in both her home life, understandably, and here at the office. Working out and eating smarter is the *best way* she knows how to do it. When things get tough, she gets tougher," Daniel says, laughing. "That woman knows how to take her stress out on a set of dumbbells, or on the stairs she often runs at lunch."

"I know! She really puts her all into her workouts," Audrey responds. "It's fun watching how intense she is, but she also seems to have so much fun with her workouts. Daniel, she *really* does enjoy it!"

Daniel goes on, "You know, that's how she got started. She and her best friend here at the office started walking the stairs at the nearby county fairgrounds stadium during lunch. The funny thing is, these two used to go out and eat—typically fast food—*every day*, for lunch, and this was a big change for them. Having each other, I believe with absolute certainty, helped them motivate each other, support each other, and hold each other accountable."

THE POWER OF SUPPORT

Thinking about her homework assignment from the last week and how supportive her family, new friends online, and Jocelyn had been the last week, Audrey asks, "Did she get a lot of support too?"

"You'd better believe it! *Everyone* here at the office has cheered her on, from day one. And she and her best friend even worked out together at lunch for a while with one of our iSatori certified trainers, a bright young man by the name of Ryan Lantzy. They both got tremendous results.

"So, wanting to push those results even further, they've since started working out with their own trainers and joined their own fitness centers, because they had different goals. But they still very much encourage each other and support each other's efforts. And, more important, they hold each other accountable by having a fun contest between them, with the rest of the company judging their results.

"Honestly, Audrey, it is something I *always* really enjoy about being the owner here…. We are all very close here and take pride in helping each other, personally and professionally, much like a family would. You will find there are a lot of caring, supportive people here. All committed to helping each other, on top of our customers, succeed—whether it's a work project or something more personal like what Jocelyn has gone through with her husband. This is the part of our company's culture I am *most* proud of."

Reflecting on her own family, Audrey feels blessed. Everyone is healthy. But when her dad got sick a few years ago, she had felt the combined work stress and personal stress and how difficult it was to get through that time. She wishes she had known then what she knows now about how exercise and eating smarter can alleviate stress to such a great degree.

"What about her family? Did she have anyone to support her?"

"Great question. And the answer is yes—Jocelyn has built a good support network of friends, family, and co-workers. You've met her granddaughter, Ashley, right?" Daniel asks.

Feeling a bit embarrassed she had forgotten Jocelyn's granddaughter name, she responds, "Oh yes, she's so sweet! She came over and ran the stairs at the fairgrounds with us a couple of days ago!"

"While I think Jocelyn would agree everyone in her family has been supportive, I am pretty certain she would say Ashley has been especially so," shares Daniel. "Every 5K race Jocelyn has run and every stair climb she competes in, since her transformation, she has Ashley by her side. They seem to have such a good time together and have built a really strong bond. As we learned in our previous session, it's vital to have a strong support system, and Jocelyn did a great job of surrounding herself with positive support—through her transformation and still today."

A DIFFICULT HOMEWORK ASSIGNMENT

Realizing she's building the same type of support system, Audrey smiles with a bit of confidence. Changing the subject, she says, "I'm sure you have a homework assignment for me, right? And I have a feeling, for some reason, this one is *not* going to be easy."

"Easy, no, sorry," answers Daniel gently. "But very much worth it—*yes*.

"That is, sometime during the next week, but before we meet again, I want you to find some time where you can be by yourself and where you can allow yourself to be completely vulnerable and honest with yourself. You need to be someplace where you won't be interrupted at all, so it can't be here at the office and likely can't be at home either—I know what it's like with small children around. Even when you think there's no chance of being interrupted, something will surely come up," says Daniel, knowingly.

Audrey agrees, blundering in, "Yeah, even in the middle of the night when everyone's supposed to be sleeping, there's still a chance of interruption!"

Daniel goes on, "So take some time away from everything and everyone—maybe on a hiking trail or at a park, or someplace that's just peaceful and quiet—like a corner of a library or a bookstore. Sit down, turn off your phone," he adds, looking at Audrey's seemingly ever-active iPhone, "and I want you to write down *your* reasons for doing this transformation for yourself.

"Remember, Audrey, your reason is *your own*. It may be unique. Or it may be something that's fairly common. But what's most important is that when you think of that reason, your why you want to change, you feel it right here," Daniel says, taking his hand and patting his chest over his heart. "It has to grab you deeply, and you realize with that reason, nothing can stop you. And I mean *nothing*.

"Write down at least one reason but no more than three. Too many reasons means they are likely not all that important. It can even be just one strong, compelling reason. Just one powerful 'why' can build incredible inspiration and momentum to pull you in the direction of your new transformation path. But, nevertheless, find a quiet place, write down your reasons, and make sure they are *your* reasons… and make darn sure they *grab you*."

Seeing the contemplative expression on Audrey's face, Daniel knows Audrey is already thinking about her reasons. "You're already coming up with something, aren't you?" he asks.

Before Audrey has a chance to respond, he continues, "It's still important to get away from everything and really let yourself dig deep into your reasons. Because I guarantee it will sustain you during any seriously difficult times in your journey."

Glancing at the clock behind Audrey, Daniel quickly gathers the pictures off the table and replaces them in the folder. "I'm sorry, Audrey, but I have to cut this one a little short today. I'm taking my daughters someplace special tonight," he adds, smiling. "So, same time next week, right?"

"Of course," answers Audrey, clearly deep in thought as she slowly places her black notebook with this week's homework assignment into her bag.

Chapter Twelve

WEEK THREE

Sitting up tall and feeling full of energy, despite the day coming to a close, Audrey writes a few notes in her little black book about her journey so far before she meets with Daniel this afternoon.

Her family has been so supportive at home, even as she's made some new recipes they'd never tried before. In fact, she couldn't believe how they happily devoured dinner last night. She had followed the recipe in iSatori's latest online newsletter, *Real Solutions for Iron Warriors*. It was healthy, loaded with vegetables and lean protein, and so tasty. Even her husband, Joe, was impressed, telling her after dinner that the meal was a definite "keeper."

Audrey had expected to have to *give up* so much on her new transformation journey, but just three weeks in, she has *gained* so much more than she imagined. Energy. Enthusiasm. And, leaning forward in her chair, she notices her clothing is starting to fit differently. *A lot differently*. Her waist band is no longer uncomfortably tight. In fact, it's getting rather loose.

Has it really been only three weeks? she thinks to herself, as she stands up and adjusts her blouse and skirt and walks out of her office. The strange thing is, she and Daniel haven't even discussed anything related to "eating" yet.

Before heading into the conference room, Audrey walks through the hall looking at the amazing "before" and "after" photos and wonders which inspiring story she'll get to hear about today.

SHARI FITNESS

She stops and pulls one off the wall to ask Daniel about. This particular photo is right near the front door and is one that has inspired Audrey since she began working there, especially when she sees the after picture says this woman is 46 years old. *She looks like she's barely in her 30's... Did she somehow discover the fountain of youth?* Audrey wonders.

Noticing the time, Audrey hustles into the conference room, just as Daniel is sitting down from writing something on the white board.

She looks up and notices the board has Lesson Number Three already written in all capital letters. It says,

LESSON #3: SET A SMART GOAL

Think big, but start small: set big, SMART, long-term transformation goals!

Audrey sets down the photos as she sits down, and before she can open her little black book to write down this week's lesson, Daniel asks...

"Are you starting to read my mind already?" To Audrey's quizzical expression, he adds, "I was going to ask you to bring Shari's photos in. Her story *perfectly* represents what we're going to talk about today."

Audrey laughs, "Well, we do spend a lot of time together during the week…

"So, please, tell me about Shari and today's Lesson," she continues, pointing to the board.

"Okay, let's not waste any time and get started," Daniel begins in his storytelling voice.

DOING IT ALL WRONG

"Nearly 10 years ago, the woman you see before you was at her lowest point in life. Although she was hitting the gym nearly every day for hours at a time, exercising 'hard,' and carefully counting every calorie she consumed, she just wasn't seeing the results she had hoped for. In fact, if anything, she was getting in *worse* shape."

"*But how is that possible?*" Audrey asks, bewildered.

"Well, unfortunately, Shari was making a few very common, but rather deadly, mistakes.

"First, she wasn't eating enough." Seeing the surprise on Audrey's face, Daniel clarifies. "I know, people are so often told, 'It's a calorie game—exercise more than you eat and you'll lose weight,' but in fact, our bodies are more sophisticated than that.

"You see, Shari wasn't eating *enough* for the energy she was putting out for her workouts, and she wasn't eating the *right* types of foods to support the changes she wanted to see in her physique, so instead of losing weight, she was actually working against her body, and doing a really great job of lowering, or slowing down, her metabolism—that's the rate the body uses stored calories for energy—to a crawl and putting her body into what's called 'starvation mode.' So the harder she tried—the less she ate, and the more she exercised—the worse she looked and felt. She wanted to give up hope but knew there had to be a better, smarter way to lose weight.

"It wasn't until Shari discovered most of what she thought she 'knew' about losing weight wasn't true and, in fact, was counterproductive to her efforts, that her *real* weight-loss successes began."

Daniel sits up straight in his chair with a wide smile on his face, as he states, "That's where our company, iSatori, came in. See, Shari had been focusing almost all of her weight-loss efforts solely on cardiovascular exercise to lose weight, and she didn't know anything about, nor the importance of, building lean muscle... But hold on, I'm getting ahead of myself..." Daniel says as he realizes Audrey is writing notes frantically in her black book.

"But this is important, *isn't it*?" she asks, looking up.

"Yes... but it's not *most* important," Daniel answers. Seeing Audrey's startled expression, he continues.

"Let me explain... Shari wanted to lose weight. She lacked self-confidence and found herself easily bullied and teased by so-called friends and some of her co-workers. Everything about her body showed she didn't feel good about herself. When she stood, her shoulders were slumped forward. She felt frumpy and walked and dressed that way. She never smiled. In fact, Shari told me once that she 'looked weak,' so it was easy for others to take advantage of her."

"What is interesting is that when Shari exercised, she felt like it was the only time of the day when she actually felt good—*about* herself and what she was doing *for* herself. But the rest of the time, she lacked energy, enthusiasm, and pretty much any joy in life. She told me that every day, she was plain and simply 'miserable.'

"But it wasn't until Shari saw a picture of herself in a bikini from a social gathering that she realized what was happening to her physically. Though her friends told her she 'looked fine,' it was obvious to her, her physical appearance was reflecting the way she felt about herself. And looking at that photo, she realized, she wanted to change. Right here, right now."

"That was Shari's *Satori* moment," Audrey blurts out cheerfully.

"Yes, that was it, Audrey. You're right," Daniel replies.

"*And do you know what she did next?* Shari took that photo and posted it on her bedroom mirror where she could see it every day when she awoke and before going to sleep at night. But she didn't just post that photo. She put a little sticky note on her photo that read '**Now Is the Time to Change!**' But, interestingly, the most significant thing Shari did that day was not just put up a photograph of herself, or the inspiring note, it was when she also wrote down some *really* ambitious goals.... What I call *SMART* goals."

"What do you mean by 'smart' goals, Daniel? How are some goals 'smarter' than others?" asks Audrey curiously.

Stretching his arms overhead and leaning back in his chair, Daniel smiles. "That's what I enjoy so much about our discussions together, Audrey. You know *exactly* the right questions to ask."

Audrey laughs at his response, knowing he's being sincere.

"So... what makes a SMART goal?" Daniel asks rhetorically.

SMART GOAL

He stands up and walks over to the board again and writes SMART in big capital letters vertically down the left hand side of the board.

Audrey grabs her pen, ready to start writing again.

"See the greatest mistake most people make when they set goals… like New Year's resolutions… is they are way too ambiguous. For instance, they set a goal to 'get fit,' or to 'lose weight.' First of all, how do you know when you achieved it? It's too vague, unclear. In fact, so much so, your brain can barely even comprehend it. And because of this, you are highly unlikely to achieve it. There is a much better, hence *smarter* way to set goals. Let me explain the process—it's actually quite simple, but again, it's a *very* powerful tool…

"First, let's start with letter S," he begins as he writes the word 'SPECIFIC' on the board. Turning to Audrey, Daniel proclaims, "You must be *specific* about what you want to achieve by creating your goals in the present tense. This is important—present tense. So, when you build a SMART goal, you need to start with something like, 'I am in the process of…' as you write your goal statement."

Seeing Audrey has finished writing and is looking back at Daniel, trying to anticipate what the M stands for, Daniel again turns toward the board. "Any guess what the M stands for?"

She responds hesitantly. "I'm not sure. Could it be something about measuring?"

"Exactly," Daniel almost bellows as he writes on the board, "MEASURABLE."

Then turning back to Audrey, he elaborates, "You see, a lot of people want to get in 'better shape.' But what does that really mean?

How do you measure that? *You can't.* Therefore, you must ensure your progress can be *measured,* by scaling your goal to a specific number. For example, it could be a body fat percentage, clothing size, scale weight, or something along those lines. So you know *exactly* when you've achieved your goal."

Again returning to the board, Daniel writes the next phrase, "ACTION ORIENTED" to the right of the letter A.

"This is one of my favorite ones. That's because in order to achieve any goal in life, whether it's losing body weight, gaining muscle, or improving your salary at work, you have to create a *list* of things *you* must do to achieve your goal. It's a lot like a 'to-do' list, only it pertains directly to the achievement of your goal. So it might be something like, 'exercise intensely at least three days a week.' 'Find a success coach' or, 'drink at least eight glasses of water each day.' Or, it can pertain to the times and/or frequency of meals you plan to eat. I normally like to see anywhere from five to ten action steps. Follow me?" Daniel asks, turning around.

Seeing Audrey's nod even as she's writing her notes, Daniel continues, writing the next word, "REALISTIC," next to the R on the board.

"This one might take some explaining. You see, you want to make certain your goals are *realistic,* so you can believe, with all your heart, you can accomplish them. But that doesn't mean you shouldn't stretch yourself. Don't be afraid to set a big, lofty goal. Just make sure it's actually doable within the time frame you've given yourself. For example, you aren't going to lose 20 pounds in a week. That's not a realistic goal. But losing 20 pounds in 12 weeks is reasonable and achievable, yet a stretch. Got it so far?"

"So far, so good," responds Audrey happily.

"Great. That leads us to the final letter, T. This one stands for TIME-SENSITIVE," Daniel says, as he writes on the board. "This is akin to… well, you know… when you prepare our monthly financials, nothing motivates us more than a deadline—a specific date we set in which we want to achieve it…"

Audrey laughs.

Returning her smile, Daniel continues, "This is where we harness the power of a deadline. Think about it, Audrey. Nothing really becomes that important or urgent to us unless we set a deadline on it. A date forces us to give it priority and sets positive pressure on us to achieve it."

Seeing Audrey set down her pen as she finishes writing down everything on the board, Daniel returns to his seat but stands behind it, placing his hands on top of his tall chair. He looks out the window momentarily as he gathers his thoughts.

"Let's return to Shari's story and how this all relates to her. As I mentioned, Shari wrote down some really SMART goals, and this was the best thing she did.

"And on top of that, *every day*, without fail, she would read her goals, several times, and she would look at that "before" picture of her body. All while she would vividly envision the body she desired by looking at a picture of a woman's body she so eagerly wanted to look like.

"Now, her goals were 'realistic.' They were *definitely* achievable, but there's no doubt she set herself some big, lofty goals. I mean, she set some really big, audacious goals, if you ask me. Her goal was that she wanted to go from where she was—frumpy, unhappy, and overweight—to looking like… and actually becoming… a professional fitness model. As you can imagine, this was ambitious, and a little bit scary, especially since she had struggled for so long to improve her physique."

Daniel went on, "Surprisingly, she almost gave up, before she started, when she discovered that in order to get in 'fitness model' shape, it meant she had to get her body fat percentage to under 15%, when she was starting at well over 30%. But, you know what? This was Shari—she was ambitious, and she wasn't going to cave in so fast. This would, in fact, become the foundation of her goal."

"As she would read her goals every day, she started to visualize her body transforming into a body she felt she would be proud of, and others would take notice of."

SMALLER STEPS

Daniel pauses and looks intently toward Audrey, and then adds, "But it gets deeper. You remember the section about 'Action Oriented'?"

Audrey nods and writes that down in her notebook.

"Well, these are basically *smaller* goals… or 'mini-goals' as I call them… which are very specific steps to achieving your goal. Basically, the steps that will take you from where you are today to where you want to be, and Shari did an incredible job of laying down a very specific set of what would become life-altering actions."

Daniel continues, "The first action step she set was to find a nutrition and exercise plan she could follow. One that *wouldn't* turn her life upside-down. And one that *wouldn't* make her count calories. So she got started looking for this plan right away. To her surprise, that very night, she went to the bookstore and looked through fitness and nutrition book after book. She finally stumbled on a book by

Shawn Phillips called *ABSolution*. She loved the photos because they helped her envision the body she wanted. And as she began reading the book, she discovered she had been a victim of some long-standing, destructive myths."

Daniel starts to lighten up and become excited as he goes on telling the story, "Then Shari set another action step of finding someone to help her learn how to properly lift weights." Smirking, Daniel adds, "Her days as the 'cardio queen' were over. She was about to discover a new, true love… one she would hold on to for the rest of her life… with resistance weight training.

"So Shari's next action step was to find and hire a personal trainer who could help her follow her new and much improved exercise plan."

"I think I'm starting to see Shari's pattern here," Audrey interrupts.

"Though Shari started with a really big goal, she broke it down into smaller, simpler action steps she could take every single day just like we do with our company goals. Each step gradually leading her in the direction and achievement of her ultimate goal," she concludes.

"But most importantly, Audrey," Daniel continues, "She took what she wrote out and she *acted on it*. Just like what you're doing. I can only share these Lessons with you. You're the one who has to take positive action."

Audrey nods realizing it really is up to her.

Daniel stands back from his chair, nearly standing on his tiptoes. "Do you know what happened to Shari…?" he asks, barely able to catch his breath, "once she started following her action steps? A mere three months later, Shari dropped her body fat in half. *In half*. She went from over 30% body fat to under 15%. She lost the flab around her hips, thighs, and on her tummy. She replaced the body fat by weight training and sculpting beautiful, new, sexy curves to her physique. She regained her energy. Her self-confidence skyrocketed. And… my favorite part… as she told me in a conversation we had afterward, '*I started smiling again. Not because of others, but because of me. How proud of myself I was and proud that others around me recognized my accomplishments and the new, happier me. It was like I gained an entirely new life!*'

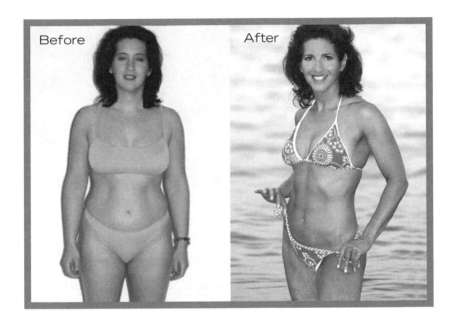

Before   After

"What is even neater than this, Audrey, was that after Shari made such an incredible transformation, her big, audacious goal came true! That is, she found her new, beautiful physique gracing the pages of the most popular health and fitness magazines, like *Oxygen* and *Fitness Rx*. She was so excited to have not only transformed her body, but she also completely transformed her life. Soon enough, she quit her lifeless cubicle day job and became a certified personal trainer. She wanted desperately to help inspire and guide others to walk in her footsteps and to experience how wonderful life can be once you make the commitment to change and follow through."

Daniel walks toward his desk and thumps his finger down on it, adding, "And today, nearly 10 years after her life-changing transformation, Shari looks even better. She runs a very popular online blog site called FitTalkNews.com, and she even wrote her own eBook called *Transformation Over 40*.

"Do you see how important this lesson is, Audrey?" Daniel peers directly into Audrey's eyes.

"She set a big, incredibly ambitious goal, and then she broke it down into small steps she could take action on. And every single year, she continues to improve. Not just her body but her entire life. And you will do the same. I know it!"

Daniel adds, with a smirk, "Rest assured, Shari's old co-workers and the people who she had called friends wouldn't recognize the powerful woman she is today. Not only does she look completely different, but she also stands tall and proud. She has an abundance of energy. In fact, I just saw Shari a few months back, and she's even leaner and more fit than the previous time I saw her. Heck, she even looks younger, and she's nearly 50 now. Needless to say, she's a force to be reckoned with," Daniel says with great delight.

Daniel quickly adds, "I wholeheartedly believe that before Shari learned the power of goal setting, there's no way she would have ever believed in herself enough to come so far. Now, she knows there is no limit to what she can accomplish, and she continues to do more and more and become better and better."

"That, Audrey," says Daniel, holding his arms out wide to indicate how much you can accomplish, "is the power of SMART goal setting!"

Returning to his seat, Daniel leans forward and writes a note down on a piece of paper, "That just reminded me," he says out loud to

Audrey. "I need to create my action steps for a little writing project I'm beginning to work on right now… Can't lose sight of that," his eyes seem to sparkle as he writes, and Audrey can see this *"little writing project"* is very important to him.

THE HOMEWORK ASSIGNMENT

Looking back at Audrey, Daniel adds, "Okay, so now it's your turn. Looking at Shari's Lesson, I'm sure you've guessed by now your homework assignment."

Audrey laughs. "I bet you're going to tell me it's time to create my own SMART goal."

"You make this too easy sometimes," he laughs back. "But you're right. Tonight, I want you to go home and write yourself out a SMART goal. Remember, that's Specific, Measurable, Action…"

"…Oriented, Realistic, and Time-Sensitive… I know, Daniel. I just spent the last 30 minutes writing them down. I didn't miss a single word," Audrey interrupts, chuckling.

Patting her notebook, she adds, "It's all here. I'll do it tonight, as soon as the kids go to sleep."

"Perfect," Daniel responds. "I'm glad we went through this one. It's very important. But I think our next Lesson is going to be *really* insightful for you…"

Audrey looks curiously at Daniel, hoping he'll elaborate and give her at least a hint. Instead, he starts to turn his chair back toward his computer, saying, "I have one more thing to finish up before I can head home for the night. I'll see you tomorrow."

Slightly disappointed, but anxious and excited, Audrey gathers her things and heads out the door.

As she climbs into her SUV, Audrey smiles, thinking about her SMART goal and imagining all she might be able to accomplish in the coming year…

Chapter Thirteen
WEEK FOUR

It's Monday, another week already, and as Audrey walks down the main hallway in the office, Daniel is walking toward her from the other direction. A few steps away, he stops and asks, "Audrey, so what did you come up with?"

Audrey, a bit confused by the open-endedness of the question replies with her own question, "What do you mean, Daniel, are you referring to this month's financial statements?"

Daniel chuckles at himself, quickly realizing he wasn't specific enough with his question, "No, I'm sorry, Audrey… I guess that was a poorly worded question, wasn't it?"

Not waiting for Audrey to reply, Daniel continues, "Actually, I mean your goals. You know, your homework assignment from our lesson last week. How did your *goals* turn out?"

Audrey appears surprised, as she wasn't expecting anything other than work-related conversations with Daniel during the middle of the day. She stutters, "Well…," and looks around to see if anyone else is in the hallway with them, "Yes… Yes, I did put together my goals."

"Are they *SMART*?" Daniel asks with sincere curiosity.

Audrey nods and replies with a smile, "Yes, they are SMART. I wrote down my goals, and they are specific, measurable, action-oriented, realistic, and … um… oh gosh, I can't remember the last part, the one that begins with the letter T…

"*Time-sensitive*. The most important part of SMART goal-setting," exclaims Samantha, the marketing manager, as she walks out of the creative graphics room, which is across the hall from Audrey's office. Audrey steps back a bit, realizing she and Daniel were standing just outside their doorway.

Samantha goes on, "Sorry, Audrey, I just couldn't help myself, and well, you looked like you could use some help on the last letter, T, of the SMART goals. I've used this goal-setting exercise for me, my husband, and even with my kids, for years now, after learning it. And I must say, it works wonderfully."

That was awfully nice of her to help me out, Audrey thinks to herself. "Thanks so much, Sam. I was stuck on that one," she says.

"Anytime, Audrey," Samantha replies, as she begins to walk away and down the hallway. Turning around and walking backward so she's facing Audrey, she adds, smiling brightly, "That's why we're here—to help each other. We're a team, *right?*"

Audrey begins to think back to her previous employer, where everyone worked in silos and protected their own jobs, not really helping one another, and were rarely all that nice to each other.

What a great place to work, Audrey thinks to herself. *No one ever treated me like this before working here.*

Daniel steps back too, away from the door and closer to Audrey's door and says, "Audrey, it sounds like you did a great job of putting together your SMART goals. How would you like to head to lunch, and go over them together now?"

Starting toward the front of the office, almost as if he expects Audrey to follow, he adds, "And, while we're there, we can cover your next lesson. Lesson Number Four. Does this work for you, instead of waiting 'til the end of the day?"

Audrey's a bit surprised Daniel would take away from their normally *very busy* Monday to go to lunch and talk about her goals and continued transformation pursuit.

She pauses, pulls out her phone to make sure she has nothing that would conflict, and then quickly replies, "Sure. Let me grab my jacket, and my notebook, and we can head out."

"Great!" then he turns back to Audrey and says, "Wait. Let me ask you a question, first…"

Daniel looks down the hallway, peering at the many pictures hanging on the walls, and says to Audrey, "Of all the before and after success stories, hanging from our walls here, which physique do you *most* admire?" To clarify, he adds, "Which person's physical transformation do you feel *most* connected to? The physique that most inspires you to achieve a similar look?"

Without hesitation, Audrey walks straight toward one picture that's a few steps behind Daniel.

"This one. Kim. I read her story in our online newsletter, *Real Solutions for Iron Warriors*, and for some reason, since then I've always connected with her," Audrey says excitedly.

"Kim Bowser," Daniel says. "I had a feeling you would choose her. I'm curious, though, what made you pick her?"

"She is beautiful. She is strong and shapely. I feel as though she is *a lot* like me. She had two kids, and it changed her. She gained a lot of weight and lost sight of herself. Just like me," Audrey says, a little sadly.

"Yes, Kim is an *extraordinary* woman. Her story is *truly* remarkable to match," Daniel says with a smile. He goes on, "And, I'm glad you picked her, because I agree, you two are similar in many ways. I can't wait to tell you her story. There's something about her that's going to surprise you, and it wasn't written in the story you read about her."

Daniel and Audrey walk out of the office front door together.

LUNCHTIME

Sitting at a small, private table in Daniel's favorite local restaurant, Blue Sky Grill, Audrey and Daniel face each other.

"I *love* this place, Audrey," Daniel says as he unfolds the napkin around his silverware. "They are always happy to accommodate your order, with any special requests. They don't charge extra for making healthy substitutions either. In fact, that's important, Audrey. Whenever you go out to eat, remember, you can order it *however* you want. *You* are paying for it. So, order your meal *exactly* how you'd like it. Don't be embarrassed. Be proud of ordering your food the way you want it, and show people you enjoy taking good care of yourself. Trust me, once you do it a couple of times, it will come naturally whenever you're ordering food at restaurants."

SMART GOALS

Getting right to the point, Daniel looks up at Audrey, "So, let's talk about your SMART goals. What are they?"

Audrey pulls out her little black notebook, where she had originally written her food journal and has been writing the transformation Lessons she's learned over the previous weeks. She flips past all of those pages and finds where she had written her goals.

"Here they are," she responds.

Audrey pulls out a pen and lightly runs it underneath the lines, where she had written her SMART goals, as if she were reading them one last time before reciting them to Daniel.

Hesitating, she finally begins to read her goal verbatim from the page, **"My goal. I am in the process of losing over 100 pounds of body weight, regaining my self-esteem, and will accomplish this within one year."**

Daniel waits, and after a few seconds of silence, finally says, "Audrey, that is an *excellent* goal. It contains all the elements of a SMART goal…"

Audrey, eagerly awaiting such approval, blurts in, "Oh good. I thought you might think it was too unrealistic."

"If you believe you can do it, which I wholeheartedly agree you can, then it's not unreasonable at all," Daniel replies, "It is perfect. It's a *big* goal, for sure, but it's reachable."

Daniel adds, "I always have to ask this… Do *you* believe you can achieve it?"

"I am *absolutely, positively* committed to achieving my transformation goal," Audrey says excitedly and goes on, almost giddy, "I know my reasons. I have already found a 'success coach' on our website at Facebook.com/iSatoriTech, and I've built an incredible group of people to support me through my lifestyle changes and this journey. I am *ready* to go! I *will* achieve my goal!"

"I *love* your enthusiasm, Audrey," Daniel says. "It's so infectious. I have *no doubt* you are going to achieve your goal. And, I can already tell, from the fact that you've been putting in place—each week—the Lessons you've learned from our talks, so I know it's only a matter of time before you achieve all you are seeking."

With all the excitement, neither of them notice the waiter standing over them, ready to set their plates of food on the table. Glancing up, Audrey jumps slightly, clearly startled, and they all laugh softly.

After getting their food, Daniel looks pointedly at Audrey's black book, saying, "I see you have more written there… your action steps I hope?"

Audrey smiles broadly. "Exactly. I've written out three steps I'm taking this week to help me accomplish my goal—including working out with Jocelyn at least three times this week and trying three new recipes from *Real Solutions for Iron Warriors.*"

"Very nice," says Daniel, smiling, as he reaches over and pours more water to refill Audrey's glass and adds, "Another great action step is to increase the amount of water you drink. It's one of the easiest and most valuable things you can do to improve your health and your weight loss!

"Now, let's talk about Kim and how you two are alike. I think there's so much you can learn from her transformation journey and there's *one lesson* in particular…"

CHANGES FOR GOOD

"With the birth of her two children, Grayson and Sophia, a mere 17 months apart, Kim's life, at the age of 35, changed more than she ever thought possible. Don't get me wrong, she loves being a mom, but her physical health deteriorated, as did her appearance, self-image, and with it, her love life.

"When I talked with Kim once, she said to me…

"'I lost sight of who I was. My inactivity, along with haphazard eating, left me watching pounds of body fat accumulate. I was depressed all the time. I didn't want to become the person I was becoming.'

"She went on, 'I was really upset at myself that I had let myself get to this point. And what's more, when I was around my kids, I always felt exhausted, and I just couldn't keep up with them, and it was killing me. Worse, both of my parents had had heart attacks, and both of my grandparents had had heart attacks, too. I was really scared I would go down that same road, so I knew if I didn't change, I was going to end up depressed, unhappy, certainly unhealthy, and maybe even dead. I was at a turning point!'"

Audrey hadn't taken a single bite of her food yet, as she was so interested in hearing Kim's story.

Daniel continues, "Fortunately, as a detective at the local police department, Kim learned about a company-sponsored physique transformation challenge, and it sparked something in her. She finally got up the courage to sign up and do it."

Daniel motions toward Audrey's plate and suggests she start eating, before her food gets cold, as he takes a couple of bites in-between telling the story. Then he continues…

"The funny thing about Kim is she didn't set any specific goals for her weight-loss transformation. She did take her before picture, however, which she dreaded doing. But, she kept her goals very vague."

"But why?" Audrey interrupts.

"I asked the same question, Audrey, and Kim confided in me that she didn't make specific goals for herself because she was afraid of failing and didn't want to set herself up for failure by setting an ambitious goal… and, as she so poignantly told me, because she had *wholeheartedly* committed to making this a permanent lifestyle change, not just a temporary change during the transformation contest period she had entered, which was for only 12 weeks."

"Could you pass the pepper?" Daniel politely asks, gesturing with his hand. "I like pepper on my eggs."

Thinking it's funny Daniel ordered a skillet with eggs for lunch, Audrey wonders if he's a bit of a mind reader when he adds, "You're probably wondering why I ordered eggs for lunch… It's my favorite meal of the day—breakfast. I could eat breakfast foods for every meal, actually. And you know what? If you think about it, almost all breakfast foods, except for bacon, are healthy for you," he says laughingly.

Audrey nods, wanting to get back to the Lesson, and comments, "So how did she do during the transformation contest?"

"Well," Daniel looks up from his plate of half-eaten food, "She won. Kim won the transformation challenge. She dropped her body fat in half. She went from over 36% body fat to under 15% body fat, during the 12 weeks. And as a result, she improved her heart health markers tremendously. She regained her energy. She even rekindled her relationship with her husband, Damon. I am so happy for her. She was the grand prize winner. But you know what was special to hear her say, *after* winning?"

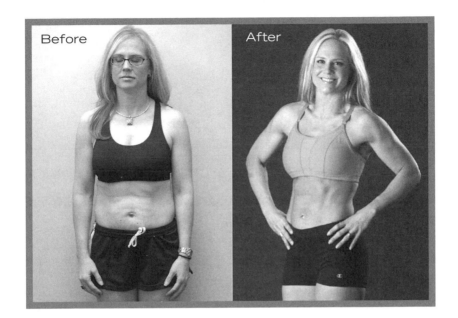

Before | After

Daniel answers his own question, "She said the transformation contest wasn't about winning any cash or prizes, it was about winning her life back!

"She now feels that, as a fit and healthy mother, she is a role model for her children. She takes them to the gym with her, and they love it. She has taught them how to read food labels and to eat smarter, and they are much more active now, too. She feels like her family is whole again, and she loves it!"

Audrey looks surprised and excited as she comments, "I am so glad for her. She sounds like a really fantastic woman, and she must have worked hard to deserve it."

Audrey takes another bite of food, realizing just how tasty her meal is, and then asks Daniel, "So, I can see how Kim and I are *a lot* alike. We are near the same age. We both have two kids. We both ate horribly. We both watched our bodies get bigger and bigger over time. We were both depressed and watching our lives spiral out of control. And sadly, we both lacked energy for our kids, our families, and our husbands. But what is the Lesson here? *Did I miss it?*"

Daniel looks away, into the distance, seemingly absent momentarily, as if he had forgotten the Lesson. He wipes his mouth with his napkin. His eyes return to Audrey's as he smiles and remarks, "I thought you'd never ask.

"I purposely left it out of Kim's story, because it didn't take place until *after* she won the transformation contest."

Audrey takes another bite and leans forward, wanting to catch every word of the Lesson.

Seeing her interest, Daniel doesn't delay and quickly continues, "Kim, her husband, and I went to dinner together one night, at a downtown restaurant to celebrate her victory in the transformation contest, and that's when she told me…"

"*What? Told you what?*" Audrey can't refrain herself from interrupting.

To which Daniel pauses and then slowly replies, "She *hated* her body."

"What?!" Audrey was perplexed and not sure she had heard Daniel correctly. Lifting her eyebrows, she adds, "Did you say…?"

"Yes," Daniel interrupts. "She hated the image she saw of her body when she looked at herself. Not just before she started, but when she finished the contest, *after* losing over half of her body fat."

Daniel continues, "I know it sounds strange, but here's what happened…"

Stunned, Audrey thinks to herself, *I don't understand how such a strong, beautiful woman could look so great and still dislike her body.*

Daniel continues, "She admitted to me that night at dinner that she hated the way she looked and wanted to look like a particular professional fitness model she knew of. When I asked her what she meant by that, she responded so eloquently, saying, *'I have a body like a boy... I have a wide waist, no hips, and thicker thighs. I'd rather look like the model on the most recent fitness magazine... she has nice curves, a thin waist, and her legs are finely sculpted.'*

"She caught me off guard. I wasn't expecting so much honesty and vulnerability from Kim. I then looked over at Damon, her husband, and he gazed back at me. Without saying a word, it was apparent this was affecting him too. Only he didn't know how to help her."

"What did you say, Daniel?" Audrey utters curiously.

"Do you remember the exercise we did, when you first started working with me, Audrey, where I asked you whether you loved yourself?"

Audrey nods.

"Well," Daniel goes on, "I left something out. That is, I left off the question of whether you loved your body, as in *your* body, *exactly as it is.*"

Daniel asks Audrey if he can look in her little black notebook. She quickly agrees, and he flips through the pages until he gets to Lesson Number Three, and turns it one more page. He then reaches out his right hand and asks Audrey, "May I?" indicating he wants to use her pen. Audrey obliges. Daniel then begins to write out the next Lesson, in her book, all in capital letters...

LESSON #4: ACCEPT YOURSELF

You must know, accept, and <u>love</u> your body, as it is.

Daniel goes back and underlines the word LOVE. "This is a very important word, Audrey. But first you must learn to *accept* your body type. See, Audrey, every body is different. Just like everyone is a different height and has different eye and hair color, and unique fingerprints, every *body* is unique, too…

"Unique in its shape, bone density, proportions of body fat, and muscle tissue."

Audrey is starting to see what Daniel is saying.

Daniel continues with a better example, "So, let's say you are Kim, and maybe you do have a thicker waist, larger sized thighs, or narrower hips than some other women. There is *nothing* wrong with this. And yes, she could change some of her shape, by losing body fat and re-shaping her muscle definition, but her basic bodily structure will not change. So, when she is looking at another female's body in the magazines, she is comparing apples to oranges. No matter how hard she tries, even after completely transforming her body, she is not going to look *exactly* like another woman whose bodily structure has a smaller waist, curvier hips, and thinner legs.

"Try as she may, Kim will *never, ever* look just like her."

Daniel continues, "And sadly, this is where many, many people go wrong—both women *and* men. They try to compare themselves to someone else's body type, only to fall short. And become disappointed when they realize that, after working out harder, eating better, and hoping to look like someone else, it's not going to turn out that way. In such disappointment comes frustration, disillusionment, and ultimately displeasure with your own physical appearance. "Fortunately, I recently spoke with Kim again just a little while ago, and she has completely transformed how she feels about her body." Pulling out his phone, Stephen adds, "Let me see if I can find her last email… Ah, here it is. This is what she emailed me after we spoke:

"'Remember when I told you I hated my body (even after the second transformation contest)? While I definitely gained more energy and self-confidence, I found I wasn't truly 'happy.' I was happiER than I had been prior to the transformation, but something was lacking, and it took me a **really** *long time to figure out what it was.*

"'I would look at other girls (figure-competitor types) and wish I looked like them. At that time, my goals were unattainable—no matter how much I thought I could out-diet and out-train my body's <u>natural</u> *shape.*

"'Because of this, I found I was always striving to be something I wasn't, which translated to me becoming increasingly more and more frustrated. I began to see the gym as a place of **<u>work</u>** *instead of a fun, healthy way to release stress and take care of my body. I didn't want to quit working out, but I wasn't happy with my training, either.*

"'I finally hit a breaking point where something had to give. A friend introduced me to CrossFit. I gave it a try, and it literally changed my way of thinking.

"'I was forced to place my focus on my actual 'FITNESS' level. I feel like a fit person now. I NEVER look in the mirror now and wish I looked differently. I LOVE the way my body looks because of what it can DO. For example, I can now do 25 pull-ups without getting off the bar. The way I feel about myself and my life now is indescribable. I feel so giddy and happy most of the time, it's disgusting.

"'I can finally say now with certainty my transformation is complete.'

"This is why it's important to understand that although it's perfectly acceptable to look at and admire other physiques, and even use someone's picture to serve as motivation or an inspiration, you should *never* try and directly compare your own body type to that of another.

"You *must, instead,* learn to accept yourself and your body, for who you are and what it is. If you're 'big-boned' or have an in-proportionate amount of fat storage around your hips, versus your waist, or whatever it is that makes you unique, then you must first learn to *understand* the differences. Then you must learn to *accept* these differences about yourself. Then, and only then, can you learn to *love* yourself."

"This is really important, Audrey," says Daniel, as he waves the pen in the air. "It's really important you learn to assess yourself, understand your differences, accept them, and then learn to love your body, *as it is*. As God gave it to you. There's a saying I recently came across that I believe to be very true: 'Exercising because you love your body versus exercising because you hate it yields very different results.'"

Audrey feels herself sinking into the chair. Although she had told herself, daily, since Daniel asked her to, that she *"loved her body,"* she didn't believe what she was saying.

The reason… she could clearly see the picture in her mind that was now taped to her refrigerator at home. It was of a younger, more slender, and *very* petite fitness model—no more than five foot tall.

Audrey suddenly realizes the mistake she has been making. This is the wrong person to compare herself to, and no matter how hard she worked to lose weight and improve her physical appearance, she would never, ever look like the young girl in that picture.

Peering closely at Audrey, Daniel asks, "What's wrong, Audrey? You look really distracted all of a sudden. Like you're somewhere else."

"I've… I've…" Audrey can't muster up enough courage to tell Daniel she has an unrealistic picture of a young model she's been using to compare herself to.

She tries to say it, but only feels herself blushing. She just can't bring herself to admit this. Pausing another moment, she finally finishes her sentence with, "I've got to find a picture of someone I can relate to. Someone who is as tall as I am… I'm five foot ten, you know…I have to find someone who is bigger boned or has a larger body frame … and someone who," she starts to laugh as she says it, "… someone who doesn't have fake breasts."

"That's right, Audrey. *That's right!*" Daniel says. "You got it. You seem to have uncovered and understand what, about your body, *is* unique, and *is* you… and you've come to appreciate it, I hope.

"Now, you can start to learn to love yourself and your body. It may not happen overnight, but if you keep saying to yourself, like I told you to do, every day—three times a day, after you look at your 'before' picture, make no mistake, you will *absolutely, positively* believe it, deep in your heart. I promise!"

Setting down Audrey's pen and taking his last bite of lunch, Daniel looks down at his watch and remarks, "Holy cow, it's been an hour and a half. Boy, time flies when you're in good company, doesn't it?!"

Audrey has heard Daniel use this saying a lot, especially around the office when in meetings and talking with employees. It always makes her feel good. Knowing he feels everyone around him in his company is "good company." It says a lot about Daniel and how much he enjoys being in the presence of his employees.

Daniel picks up his napkin from his lap, wipes his mouth, and places it neatly beside his plate, before saying, "Audrey, here's your homework…"

Audrey reaches for her pen and her black book. But before she can turn to a new page, Daniel blurts…

"You don't need to write this down. I could hardly imagine you'd forget what I'm about to say, especially after today's conversation."

HOMEWORK ASSIGNMENT

Daniel continues, "That is, for your homework, I'd like you to visit a Barnes & Noble bookstore tonight… with your kids or by yourself… flip through the magazines until you find a physique you feel you *really* connect with. One, as we've learned, that's similar to *your own body's* uniqueness.

Daniel proceeds to signal to the waiter that he's ready for the check, "It may take you awhile to find someone in those magazines, but you will. And, trust me, it will be well worth it. Then, I'd like you to take that picture and hang it up on your refrigerator. What do you think? Can you do that?"

Audrey looks at Daniel with a guilty smirk on her face, as she begins to chuckle and mutters, "I can do that. Not a problem. I'm actually looking forward to this exercise. It will be fun."

"Great. Now, let's get back to the office and finish our day," Daniel says even as he's walking toward the door, checking his phone for any urgent phone calls, texts, or emails.

As they exit the restaurant, Daniel looks up and waves goodbye to the owner, all the while Audrey's thinking to herself about the picture she already has hanging on her refrigerator that desperately needs to be replaced…

Chapter Fourteen
WEEK FIVE

Audrey's more eager today than on the past four Mondays. Though she doesn't know why, the butterflies in her stomach are a pretty good indicator she's overly anxious and excited about her meeting with Daniel today.

By already putting the first four Lessons to practice, she's amazed at the way she feels—more vibrant, alive, and full of optimism. She's even more amazed at the improvements she's already seen in her physique. Most of all, Audrey's *filled* with hope.

She wonders what her Lesson will be today.

As she walks down the hallway toward Daniel's office, Leroy, the company's chief financial officer and her boss, comes out of his office, about to leave for the night, and intercepts her.

"Audrey?" he politely asks with his strapping Texas accent, "Are you staying late again tonight?"

Unprepared for the question, Audrey isn't exactly sure how to answer Leroy, since she wasn't going to talk with Daniel about work-related stuff, so she hesitates. Not one to tell a lie, she keeps her answer short, "*Um... well, yes... I have some things to cover with Daniel.*"

As Leroy turns to close his door behind him, he notices the picture on the wall outside his office door hanging crooked. He reaches out to straighten it, and as he does, he remarks, "Boy oh boy, this one has always been my favorite. She made such an incredible transformation and has become such an inspiration to so many people!"

"What's her name?" Audrey quickly asks.

"Carla," Leroy replies, "Carla Iansiti, from Lansing, Michigan."

"She lost 77 pounds," adds Daniel, finishing Leroy's sentence.

Leroy replies back in the most affectionate tone, "And her pictures look like two *completely* different women. If I didn't know her personally, I'm not sure I'd believe it. But I'll tell you, her transformation is real, and that lady is now as pretty as a speckled pup."

Daniel and Audrey laugh at Leroy's comment. They both know him well enough to know he means that comment with sincere affection.

Daniel continues, "She sure is a beautiful woman. And her transformation on the outside is a mere reflection of the transformation that took place on the inside. She is a beautiful person, inside *and* out."

"Well, goodnight, ya'll. I'll see you bright and early tomorrow," Leroy quaintly signs off to Daniel and Audrey by mimicking the tipping of his hat to the both of them.

"Good night, Leroy," Daniel and Audrey say almost in unison.

"Well, Audrey, are you ready?" Daniel asks as he turns to walk back toward his office.

"Of course… *But…*" Audrey pauses.

"But what?" Daniel asks.

Audrey smiles and replies, inquisitively, "Shouldn't we take Carla's before and after pictures with us?"

Daniel smiles and embarrassingly replies, "Oh yes," turning to take Carla's pictures off the wall. "Thanks for remembering."

AUDREY'S MIRROR IMAGE

Sitting in Daniel's office, he notices Audrey looking closely at Carla's picture, as he comments, "Actually, Carla reminds me a lot of you, Audrey. You two are similar in many ways."

Interrupting Daniel, she asks, "In what way… *I mean…* Carla looks like a strong and confident woman… I bet it came easy for her to lose all that weight… She didn't have to struggle that much at all, did she?" Audrey's so excited to hear Carla's story, she can barely get the words out.

"Actually, it was quite the opposite, Audrey. Carla struggled from a very early age with her weight. Much like you, she attempted diet after diet, only to find herself and her body weight continually yo-yoing. Her body image was always very poor, as far back as she could remember," Daniel shares.

"One time, during a very long and surprisingly honest conversation with Carla, she admitted to me some personal things that astounded me. I really felt for her. She said…

"'I've always struggled with my weight, even when I was a child. In fact, I remember when I was in the 5th grade, and I weighed 120 pounds already, a kid called me fat in front of the class, and everyone laughed out loud. My life was never the same again. My view of myself was always positive, but when I would look in the mirror, the reality of seeing myself as 'fat' would set in. I would start saying to myself how I'm gross, and obese, and no one would ever like me, let alone love me. I became depressed at an early age. From as far back as I can remember, all I have ever done is worry about my weight and how it makes me feel so horrible about myself. And no matter what I've done to lose weight, nothing has worked… Nothing!'"

Continuing with her story, Daniel adds, "When Carla turned 40, she weighed her heaviest at 262 pounds and was a size 22. The excessive weight was causing chronic pain in her back and knees. She felt completely helpless and lost."

Looking at Audrey compassionately, Daniel says to her, "And this is where you and Carla are so much alike. Like you, she tried *every* conceivable way to lose weight, only to fail, and worse, continue to unwillingly gain weight."

THIS TIME… THIS TIME…

Daniel then leans back into his chair, getting comfortable to settle in and tell Audrey a humorous story to illustrate his point…

"Much like the little bumblebee, Barry Benson, played by Jerry Seinfeld in the *Bee Movie*, when he accidentally got locked in the apartment window of Vanessa Bloom, played by Renee Zellwegger. He kept trying to fly out, not realizing it was a closed glass window. As he attempts to fly out, he vigorously flies and bumps into the closed window, though he keeps trying and saying to himself, '*this time, this time, this time, this time.*' Finally, after countless failed attempts, he finally gives up and is left hopelessly sitting on the windowsill.

"Carla, after trying diet after diet after diet… and failing time and time and time again… *certainly* was left wondering if she'd ever lose the weight. She kept trying and trying and somehow, she remained positive most of the time, believing she would find the solution eventually."

"What else did she try, besides dieting?" asks Audrey curiously.

"Pretty much everything. And I mean *everything*." Daniel proceeds to rattle off what seems like an endless list…

"She enrolled in a local medical weight-loss clinic, where she ate their prescribed pre-packaged foods that she said tasted like cardboard but found she was more informed than the people who worked there and hated the embarrassing weigh-ins.

"She bought into a program from Jenny Craig, but felt it was too expensive and she didn't even make it home before she was filled with guilt about eating out of a box and returned it.

"She joined countless gyms and even worked at a gym to be around healthy people and learn their 'tricks.'

"She purchased a BodyBugg, and while it helped count calories, it didn't help her determine which foods were actually healthy.

"She subscribed to online weight-loss websites and health publications, in the hope she would find a source of information to help her.

"Her doctor prescribed her several different prescription-strength diet pills, which didn't live up to their claims and only made her feel sick to her stomach.

"And over the years, she followed pretty much every fad diet that came along, leaving her feeling deprived and malnourished.

"It's also important to understand that Carla was no couch potato. Despite the extra weight she carried most of her life, she loved to play sports, ride bikes, and was a great athlete. She tried to work through her pain, but when it got to be too much, she was left even more confused and frustrated. She would end up stopping but then would always start again, believing 'this time' would be different.

"Luckily, her *final* attempt… well, it became her 'Satori' moment. This is what changed Carla's path, forever…"

ENOUGH WAS ENOUGH

Sitting up straighter, Audrey scoots her chair closer to Daniel's desk, indicating she doesn't want to miss one word of this part of Carla's story and her soon-to-be-learned lesson.

"Carla had finally decided *enough was enough*, so she went to a seminar for people who wanted to undergo bariatric surgery. This, she felt, was her last resort. She arrived early at the event, well before anyone else, but once others started to arrive, she couldn't help but notice the health of many of them. Clearly, as she put it, 'it was a live or die situation for them.' She didn't feel she belonged there, but worried if she didn't figure out her eating habits and lose that unhealthy weight she was carrying around, she would be in their same predicament. Then, *the* moment came… the person hosting the meeting told Carla that to qualify for their bariatric surgery, she needed to weigh at least 270 pounds, and if she wanted to do it, she would have to gain *more* weight to meet their qualifications. (She weighed 262 pounds.)

"Frustrated beyond belief, she immediately left, feeling hopeless once again. Dejectedly, before she even reached her car, she burst into tears. She called her husband to tell him the story of what had happened at the seminar and could barcly talk because she was crying so hard.

"That's when it set in. She didn't know where to turn. She felt like her world was ending, and she had nowhere else to go. She was deeply depressed. And worse, felt like no one, at this point, could help her. She thought, 'That's it. I was made fat, and I'm going to stay fat.' But there was a little voice in her head that said different. Something wasn't right. She felt good on the inside most of the time, so why not on the outside?

"It was in this *very* moment of self-reflection she realized she wasn't going to find her solution—to lose weight, to become healthier, to become happier—in any *one thing*, externally. Not in a magazine article. Not in a pill. Not in a clinic. Not in a pre-packaged food. And, surely not in a new weight-loss gimmick sold on TV. She became immediately conscious that instead she needed to look *internally*. Her 'moment of clarity' struck."

LOOKING THROUGH A NEW LENS

"She needed to change the way she looked at things. She needed to change the way she thought about food and her approach to eating. In other words, to lose the weight, *once and for all*, she would need to change *her* association to food and understand that losing weight is a journey… a lifelong approach to eating smarter that starts from the *inside*."

Daniel abruptly sits up in his chair, uncrosses his legs, and plants his feet firmly on the floor and leans forward as he continues to gain excitement telling Carla's story, "It was the next day Carla's husband told her about this company—*our* company, in fact—that he was absolutely, positively convinced could help her.

"See, Carla's husband had seen a program on a well-known doctor's television show, where he learned about a new way of eating. So he went to a nearby health-food store to gather some more information about the company. He came home and told her all about it. He was *so* excited because, for some strange reason, he knew this was *it* for her. This company… our company… would help her *finally* transform from the inside out and make lasting changes.

"Carla immediately began doing some research through our social media site on the web. It was there she discovered a new online community of friends who would help her completely transform her life, for the better, forever."

Standing suddenly, Daniel begins to walk toward the Japanese plaque on the wall. Pointing to it, he says, "That's it, Audrey, Lesson Number Five, and the most important…"

THE NEXT LESSON

"Stop looking to outside solutions to solve your weight problems," Audrey blurts out, cutting Daniel short.

"Wow! Close. *Very* close, Audrey," Daniel replies, smiling.

He proceeds to pick up his favorite blue marker and write on the white board, beneath Lesson Number Four:

LESSON #5: LOOK INWARD

To help guide your transformation journey to lasting weight loss, you must no longer look outward, and instead look inward.

As Audrey carefully writes it down in her black book, Daniel continues to tell her, "If not for this moment in her life—to her looking *inside* herself, to make the decision to commit herself to a long-term approach to eating smarter and losing weight, and stop leaving her fate in the hands of some *thing* or some *person*, she wouldn't be where she is today… a renewed, beautiful, remarkable, healthier woman.

"As you can see, from the before and after pictures you're holding of Carla, she transformed how she looks on the outside *and* how that reflects the way she feels about herself can be seen in her confident energy in her 'after' picture."

Daniel went on, "And what's even more incredible about her is that nearly two years after her remarkable transformation, I have received additional photographs from Carla. She continues to get lighter and lighter, and look better and better… and every time I talk with her, she's happier and happier about herself and her life.

"But, make no mistake, Audrey, it all started by her looking *inward*. And this may be the most critical lesson, in and of itself, to committing yourself to this lifelong, rewarding journey.

Daniel turns and looks out the window. He clears his throat and states, "That's your fifth Lesson, and a *really* essential one, especially considering how closely I believe you resemble Carla and her lifelong challenges with her body and weight."

Audrey feels like she's has gotten to know Daniel well enough, so she's comfortable asking him, "*Why…*" then hesitating for a moment, and asks, "Why are you getting choked up?"

Daniel again clears his throat and turns back to Audrey, "Because, Audrey… because Carla reminds me so much of *you* and the challenges and painful struggles you've dealt with all your life. And, *damn it*, if she can do it, so *can you!*"

Daniel walks toward Audrey and gently places his hand on her shoulder, adding, "I know you can succeed too, Audrey, and I *wholeheartedly* believe you will. You *will* succeed and finally achieve the body and life you've always wanted and deserve. And you know, I can already see it happening to you. It's only a matter of time now before you see it yourself. So I guess I got a little choked up knowing that."

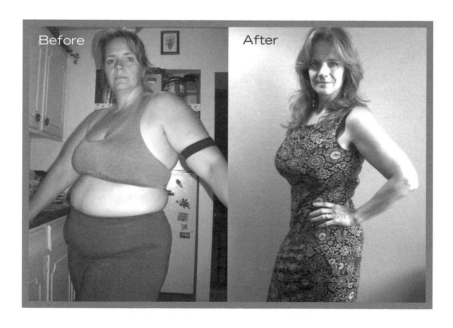

Daniel squeezes Audrey's shoulder and then returns to his chair and sits back down, as he tells what remained of Carla's extraordinary story, "I'm happy to tell you Carla is celebrating her second anniversary at her new weight. She has slimmed down to 185 pounds—the lightest she has weighed in her entire adult life. In total, she lost over 77 pounds, is down to a size 10, and can now get out of bed without taking any medications or having a stiff back or knees. And the best part is that Carla told me she feels *absolutely* comfortable in her new body, and her husband, who has been her greatest supporter all along, and loved her no matter what her size was, says she looks 'downright sexy!'"

BEING ACCOUNTABLE

"What's even more exciting to me is Carla has become one of our most sought-after transformation 'success coaches' in our online community at iSatori.com. There she connects with many women and men who, like her, were challenged their entire lives with yo-yo diets and fluctuating body weight. She inspires them. She encourages them. She answers their questions, daily. And especially important, she holds them accountable.

"See, Carla admitted to me that when she was first starting her weight-loss transformation with us, and all during the first year, she would post a comment daily…" seeing Audrey's surprised look, Daniel emphasizes, "Yes, *daily* in our online community, just to keep herself accountable. And, I must say, it worked out marvelously well for her."

Daniel leans back again, but looks more serious, as he continues, "Interestingly, though, when I asked Carla what the most important thing she did during her transformation journey was, she told me this:

"Journaling everything I ate was a daily exercise I attribute much of my success to. Not a food journal necessarily. I didn't jot down every single calorie I ate. Rather, I kept notes in my journal of which foods made me feel good and which foods made me feel bad. Through this exercise, I now understand how food can make you feel physically and emotionally—up or down. Over time, I learned that certain foods make me feel bloated or sluggish and even tired. And other foods give me energy and make me feel so much more vibrant. I learned that when I feed myself more frequently throughout the day with fresh foods and drink plenty of water, I feel more alert and alive. I have developed a lifestyle to eat smarter that, thankfully, my entire family now benefits from. Unlike diets, where no one else in your household, except maybe your spouse, can follow your same diet, making a lifestyle choice to simply eat smarter foods your whole family can enjoy is so much more fun and rewarding."

NOT A DIET

"What does Carla typically eat… what does her diet … oops, I mean, what does her way of eating look like now?" Audrey interjects, as Daniel comes to a close.

"Good, I'm glad you caught yourself. It's not a diet. It's a lifestyle," Daniel says with a chuckle.

He goes on to answer her, "Actually, that's a great question, Audrey. Because I knew you and I would be covering this very topic, I asked Carla to send me an email with her daily eating habits written out."

Daniel proceeds to pull out a single printed piece of paper. Before he begins to read it, he prefaces, "A typical day of eating for Carla, these days, looks something like this…

"**Upon waking up**: She starts her day with a tall glass of water; followed by a cup of hot water with fresh squeezed lemons. This helps aid in digestion and cleanses the body in the morning.

"**At 7:00,** she starts her day with an Eat-Smart® nutritional meal-replacement shake. As you know, it's very simple to make: you just add water, ice cubes, and the Eat-Smart powder into a blender, and mix it up. It tastes like a milkshake. Oftentimes she adds some fresh fruit like strawberries or blueberries.

"**Around 8:00,** she has a cup of coffee with a packet of Splenda to sweeten it.

"**For a mid-day snack, around 10:00**, she has an apple—golden delicious is her favorite—and a handful of raw unroasted nuts, with a piece of melba toast.

"**Lunch is her biggest meal of the day, and she eats it around half past noon.** She usually eats a hearty salad, with lots of mixed greens, piles on carrots, cucumbers, corn, tomatoes, broccoli, and sprinkles on some pine nuts, and red grapes for added flavor. She uses a homemade dressing made with virgin olive oil, flax seed oil, and balsamic vinegar. She adds a sliced chicken breast to her salad to complete the meal. Sometimes she will also have a slice of whole-grain bread with lunch.

"**Her midday snack, around 3:00,** when most people are reaching for Coke and a Snicker's bar, she insists on something smarter and healthier. She's a big advocate of packing foods to bring with her, so she doesn't make poor choices. She will usually eat a small Greek yogurt, sliced fruit, with some chopped nuts or muesli cereal mixed in. If she doesn't have any of these foods on hand, while at work, she will opt to snack on something similar to her mid-morning snack—like a piece of fruit or a cup of mixed berries, an orange or a grapefruit, along with a handful of nuts. If neither of these options are readily available, she'll munch on an Eat-Smart nutritional bar. These are delicious, healthy protein bars that keep you feeling fuller for longer than other bars because they contain extra protein and fiber.

"**She normally prepares dinner for her family around 6:00** after she comes home from work, where she makes an array of delicious meals, like chicken and veggie stir fries, broiled salmon, grilled chicken, or lentil soups, coupled with vegetable dishes that are filling and tasty. She always stresses the importance of eating lots of protein along with plenty of fresh vegetables, and limits the carbohydrates to whole-grains like brown or wild rice, sweet potatoes or yams, and quinoa.

"**For dessert, *yes dessert*,**" Daniel smiles as he sees Audrey's head snap up from the notes she's taking. "**Around 8:00 or 9:00,** Carla makes herself a scrumptious Eat-Smart nutritional pudding. Again, it's so easy to make: she simply adds one scoop of Chocolate-Chocolate Chip Eat-Smart powder to a half a cup of water, stirs thoroughly, and lets it chill in the refrigerator for about 10 to 15 minutes, and it tastes a lot like JELL-O chocolate pudding—only it's *healthy* for you!

"And throughout the day, and with every meal, she drinks tall glasses of water. In all, she drinks about 8 to 10 glasses of water a day, and she keeps plenty of vegetables and fruits and nuts around for snacking.

"She avoids any fast-food places. In fact, she says she and her husband Tom haven't had any fast food in over five years. Since you and I have young children, we know that can be difficult. So I personally choose 'fast casual' restaurants that have smarter food choices, like Chick-Fil-A, Chipotle, or Jamba-Juice, where I can ensure my family is getting good, wholesome food choices.

"As you can see, Audrey, her daily eating habits are actually quite simple. You'll notice, however, there is a theme to her eating…

"First… *frequency throughout the day*, for a total of five meals or snacks.

"Second… she always, always, always *includes protein, along with veggies or berries, in each meal or snack.*

"Third… she drinks plenty of water throughout the day.

"And finally, she goes for homemade convenience, whenever she can, over preparing intricate, time-consuming meals or eating out."

"There doesn't seem to be anything *too* terribly difficult or complex about her eating habits," Audrey says as if she's waiting for Daniel to spring something else on her.

"No, not at all," Daniel responds enthusiastically. "Like I said, it's not a diet; it's a lifestyle. It's a brand new association with food. Eating to live, not living to eat. It's a lifelong approach to eating smarter. Carla has told me she's not afraid of food anymore. She just focuses on eating *real* food and avoids virtually anything boxed or that claims its low fat or sugar free. It's a way she can enjoy eating with her entire family."

Daniel glances over at the clock on his desk and almost falls out of his chair, "Holy cow, it's almost 6:30. It's time to get you out of here to your kids, and I'd better get home, too."

THE NEXT HOMEWORK ASSIGNMENT

"What's my homework assignment tonight?" Audrey eagerly asks before beginning to pack up her notes.

"Well, it has to do with your eating," Daniel replies.

"You've already done a great job of writing down what you ate for the first three days we worked together. Remember that… In your little black book?"

Audrey nods.

Daniel adds, "Tonight, I'd like you to go home and plan out your eating for the next week. That is, I'd like you to write a daily eating plan journal, starting from the time you wake up to the time you go to bed. And be sure to include what you plan to drink as well. I suggest you simply put in the times of the day, and then fill in what you plan to eat at each time. This way you'll be able to plan the entire day, for all of your meals and snacks. Once you've done this for one day, go ahead and fill out another six days of meal plans for a total of seven days."

Audrey starts to shuffle her belongings together.

Daniel concludes, "If you get confused, or frustrated for ideas at any point, I'd encourage you to go online to our website, at iSatori.com, and look at the recipes. I think you'll find plenty of inspiration there to help you fill in each and every meal and snack.

"Oh, and I almost forgot, make sure your meals, like supper, when you are home, are those you can enjoy with your *entire* family. Okay?"

"Sure thing," Audrey replies, as she quickly writes down the homework instructions. "I can do that tonight. Not a problem at all. Actually, I am quite excited about this assignment, because I've already been exploring around our online community, making lots of new friends, and picking up some incredibly healthy new recipes that are really delicious! And on top of that, Jocelyn has been showing me how to prepare healthier lunches, after our midday workouts."

Audrey picks her keys out of her purse and rushes off.

But before getting out of the doorway, she stops, turns, and says to Daniel, "Thank you, Daniel. *Thank you* for doing this with me. It means a lot to me, and I was happy to hear today that you believe in me. That means a great deal to me. I feel a lot like Carla must have… at this point, when she felt like this was it—this was her time to change, for the better and forever. I feel that same way *right now*."

Daniel looks at Audrey with a big smile but doesn't say a word.

Audrey turns and walks out, calling down the hallway, "Have a good night."

Chapter Fifteen

WEEK SIX

Audrey looks at her watch and is surprised to see it's 5:15 p.m. She's late. Her usual Monday appointment with Daniel was supposed to start 15 minutes ago. She grabs her black book, a pen, and her phone and rushes to Daniel's office.

It's been raining all day, and as Audrey walks into Daniel's office, she notices how much colder it is than hers. Out of breath, she starts to explain, "Daniel, I'm sorry…" before she sees he's not sitting in his chair, or anywhere else in his office.

Suddenly, Daniel startles her from behind. "Looking for me, Audrey?" Daniel asks with a wink.

Audrey turns around to notice he's carrying a picture frame in his hands. "Sorry I'm late…" she again starts to say.

"It's fine. I was running late, too. I just had time to go out into the hallway and find the before and after pictures of the story we're going to talk about today."

"Who is it?" Audrey asks curiously, as she tries to peek at the picture.

"One of the most remarkable transformations I have ever been lucky enough to witness. Tony Martinez. He lost over 60 pounds and 11 inches off his waist, in the first few months of his lifestyle change," Daniel answers.

"Over 60 pounds in a few months?!" Audrey exclaims. "Is that possible?"

"Yeah, hard to believe, isn't it?" Daniel responds. "But he did it—he completely transformed himself, on the inside *and* outside, in just a few short months, with one simple trick."

A trick? Audrey thinks to herself.

"Not really a trick, but rather one particular *Lesson* Tony took to heart and followed religiously," Daniel responds, knowing Audrey was wondering what "trick" he was referring to.

Daniel continues, "And the best part is, Tony has kept improving his physique more and more over the years. In fact, the last time I saw Tony, he told me he recently went to a family reunion where many of his family members who hadn't seen him for several years honestly didn't even recognize him."

As Daniel points to Tony's picture, he adds, "He had changed that much!"

"That's so incredible," Audrey exclaims.

"So what was the trick...or, ummm... rather, *the Lesson* he paid special attention to?" she asks anxiously.

"Well, Audrey, that's what we are going to talk about today. You probably want to sit down for this one, because I have a hunch you might not want to hear what I'm about to say..."

"Why's that?" Audrey interrupts.

"Because this is *the* Lesson that separates those who completely... and I mean *completely*... transform their physical appearance from those who make only a small change physically.

"And make no mistake about it, Audrey, what is even more amazing is that... and I've seen it over and over again throughout the years... this *one* Lesson provides *so many more* benefits than just your physical changes; that is, it will improve literally *all* other parts of your health, too!"

Anxious to hear Tony's story and learn this week's Lesson, Audrey quickly sits down just as Daniel does, before they get on their way...

TONY THE PIZZA GUY

"Tony loved pizza. He also loved donuts, French fries, and sitting on the couch. So much so that on the last visit he made for a 'checkup,' his doctor told him he needed to start using a prescription blood-thinner medication for his high blood pressure; his asthma was the worst it had ever been; he was now borderline diabetic; and if he didn't start eating better and working out, he would become yet another poor health statistic, or worse, he'd die.

"Tony, a police officer, had fallen into the stereotype of how a policeman would wind up—after years of eating donuts for breakfast, a couple of pieces of pizza for lunch, and munching on bags of chips combined with drinking sugared soda pops throughout the day, while on his patrol rides. Tony found himself inactive, because he was always so tired. The sum of these poor decisions over the years ballooned his weight up to 255 pounds and pushed his waist out to 44 inches, even though he stood at only five foot seven inches tall.

"When I met Tony, prior to his transformation, he told me this, *'All I do is sleep all the time. I am so depressed. I'm not motivated to do anything. My job… my marriage… my health are suffering dramatically because of my bad habits. I hate the way I look and the way I feel. I want so desperately to get out of this horrible place I'm in, physically. But I don't know what to do.'*

"In that very moment… *his 'Satori' moment*… I knew Tony was ready for change. He was not happy with himself, physically *or* spiritually. He had strong, compelling reasons to change. He knew his wife and fellow officers would support him. He just needed to set some smart goals, and he needed a clear plan and path. He was ready for help, and I felt it was my responsibility… and my privilege… to provide him with the answers to make that change.

"See, I've always felt that police officers are our community's greatest role models. When I was younger, they, along with members of the armed forces, were like superheroes to me. I've always looked up to them. They are supposed to be fit and healthy. Able to chase down the 'bad guys' and keep us safe. And sadly, Tony had found himself far from this picture of perfect physical health and heroism.

"So we decided to meet for coffee and discuss what type of changes he wanted to make. Before we met, I had asked Tony to come prepared with his goals written out—what he wanted to achieve from our conversation.

"We met at a nearby Barnes & Noble bookstore with a Starbucks inside. Tony told me his goal was to make the most impressive transformation, *and the fastest*, I had ever seen. At first, I was taken aback by his boldness and ambition. He then told me his goal was to get below 200 pounds and reduce his waist by at least 10 inches, in less than 10 weeks. And that wasn't all...

"He then looked squarely into my eyes and said to me, 'I want your secret to making fast changes, and I mean fast. I'm serious about this, Daniel!'"

"What did you say to him?" Audrey blurts out, with sincere curiosity.

"This is where it gets *really* interesting, Audrey..." Daniel replies. "Tony wasn't ready for my reply, that's for sure."

THE UNEXPECTED

"'Tony,' I replied with a bit of nervousness in my voice, after his stern statement, knowing my reply to him wouldn't be what he was hoping to hear. 'I appreciate your ambitious goals. And I admire your willingness and desire to change. It's important to remember, though, the type of change I teach is *lasting* change. *Not* a quick fix. They are Lessons that create new lifestyle habits that endure. They are intended to last a lifetime, well beyond your initial weight loss.'

"'I get that,' Tony replied. 'I respect it, truly I do. But, I want you to show me your secrets... the secrets I've seen in other transformations before me, which happened so quickly.'

"That's when I leaned back in the chair and decided it was time to share my 'secrets' with Tony. So with a smile on my face, I responded, 'Tony, the secret is... well... the secret is there are *no* secrets. There is no *one thing* that will help you. You see, it's *everything*. It's putting into practice *everything* I am willing to share with you and applying it consistently over time. But if you truly think there is a *secret*, then you've come to the wrong person.'

"Tony didn't look too happy to hear my response. That's when I decided to make a deal with him.

"'What I can tell you, Tony, however, is if you promise me you will take what you learn from me… and make your new lifestyle changes carry on *well beyond* your initial transformation… I will provide you with a single lesson that will help you make a rapid transformation in your physical shape.'

"Tony agreed, so I went on.

"'Tony,' I said to him, 'along with all the other Lessons you are going to put into practice, I am going to provide you with one Lesson in particular that is going to help you make exceptionally fast progress. It's an exercise program that will help you improve your physical appearance, fast. It's a very challenging workout program, and the most technically sound I have ever created. And make no mistake about it, my friend, when you have completed it, you will have made more changes in your physical shape than you could have ever imagined. In fact, my hunch is, based on my experience of working with others much like you, you'll experience more changes in one month than most people do after years of struggling.'

"Tony looked excited and asked me to show him the workout program. He was eager to try it and willing to get started right away.

"'First, Tony,' I explained, 'There is something really important you should know. The reason I am stressing the importance of physical exercise, specifically weight training combined with cardiovascular exercise, is because doing these together is the *only* way to re-shape your body. It's the only way to strengthen, buildup, and reshape your muscular frame. And in doing so, it's the only way to truly speed up your metabolism—the rate at which your body uses excess body fat for energy. It's the only way to strengthen your bones and skeletal structure. It's the only way to alleviate stress, anxiety, and even naturally cure depression. And, it's the only way to strengthen your heart—the largest and most important muscle in our bodies.

"'See, there is so much scientific evidence—studies published in peer-reviewed scientific journals and real-world empirical data—that shows whether you move a little, or exercise intensely, it's the only way to trade in unhealthy, unshapely body fat for lean, shapely muscle tissue and markedly improve all of these other health statistics I just mentioned. Which means it's the only way to truly change the way you look. And, what's more, it will provide you with so many more healthy benefits as well as change the way you feel too.'

"Tony looked up at me with a hint of desperation on his face and said, 'Daniel, I've got to admit. I'm a bit nervous.'

"'Why is that?' I asked.

"'Because… well, to be honest, when I was in the marines, I worked out pretty religiously, and after I got out and joined the police force, my partner died, and since then, I haven't stepped foot in the gym. That was nearly seven years ago. And worse, I hate to admit it, but I really don't like working out any more. In fact, I dread it.'

"'It's okay, Tony,' I assured him. 'Most people feel the same way you do. You are certainly not alone. But trust me, once you get started working out again, seeing how quickly the changes in your body happen, you will not want to stop.'

"I provided Tony with an exercise program that is actually one I spent several years creating and that I follow myself. It's affectionately called the '5-4-3-2-1 workout success system.' I call it that because it's essentially a fail-proof workout plan—a countdown to your success. It's like a paint-by-numbers system. You simply follow along and are basically guaranteed to see results.

"There are three keys to the workouts that are the primary reasons this system is so successful, once you follow it," Daniel explains. "First, the workouts must change daily. This is important, Audrey, because most people get tired of doing the same exercises, in the same order, day after day. By changing it up so frequently, not only do you get a fresh, new workout each day, but also because of this, your body can never adapt or get used to the workouts, so you are better able to experience continuous improvements. The second key is the workouts need to be intense. This means they get your heart rate up and keep you moving, *consistently* throughout the workouts. Interestingly, not only does this keep you more motivated during your workout, it also makes the time go by faster. As a result, you burn more calories during *and after* the workout. The third, and final, key to the workouts is they must combine *both* weight-training and cardiovascular exercises. These are equally important—resistance weight training *and* cardiovascular exercise. See, contrary to common belief, one without the other doesn't produce nearly the same results. They are directly linked.

"Let me explain how the workouts are structured… "

CROSSING THE FINISH LINE

Before Daniel can finish his sentence, Audrey asks, "So, how did Tony do, once he got started?" eager to find out.

"I'm pleased to say… and must admit… I was quite astonished by Tony's progress," Daniel replies with excitement building in his voice. "Tony beat his goals… actually he *crushed* his goals. He dropped his weight below 200 pounds. To be exact, when he started, he weighed a hefty 250 pounds, and afterward, he weighed in at 187 pounds."

"That means he lost…" she quickly does the math her in head… "He lost 63 pounds! Wow, that's incredible—almost unbelievable!" Audrey interjects.

"Yes, he did, he lost 63 pounds of ugly, unhealthy body fat. Isn't that amazing? And on top of that, Tony lost 11 inches off his waist, dropping his waist size from a 44 down to 33.

"For the first time since his teenage years, Tony was able to see his abdominal muscles… he had developed the admired six-pack. And what's more, when he went back to see his doctor, he was amazed at how much his health markers had improved."

Daniel starts to get more excited as he continues, "The best part,

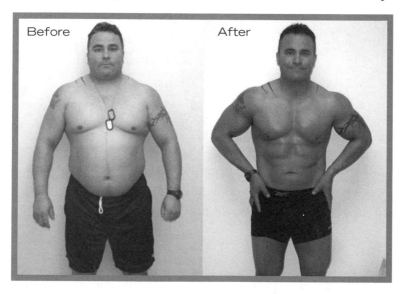

and most surprising to me, Audrey, is that he did this in only nine weeks. *Nine weeks.* This is simply remarkable!"

Daniel concludes, "You know, I've been helping people make transformations and lose weight for nearly 20 years now, but I have to say, Audrey, until Tony, I had yet to see anyone lose weight, and reshape their body, so rapidly. Tony looked like a completely different person, after only nine weeks of eating smart and working out intensely."

Daniel points at Tony's picture and remarks, "Just look at his pictures. They say it all. In his before picture, he looks very unhappy and unhealthy. And then when you look at his after pictures, you see how much happier and healthier he looks. *I love that.* That is why we do what we do here at our company. I absolutely *love* seeing people make such incredible physical changes and the difference it makes to their expressions in their after pictures. It's a reflection of their renewed spirit. You can see... you can see it in their spirit... the physical transformation that takes place on the outside. It is merely a reflection of the transformation that takes place on the inside.

"Afterward, Tony and I saw each other when he came up to visit me here at the office. He told me, 'This transformation changed my personality, and frankly, my entire outlook on life. I am no longer grumpy or depressed. My attitude is always positive in everything I do. It has affected pretty much all parts of my life... and made me better at my job, my marriage, and in all of my interactions with people every day. I feel like I have the confidence to accomplish anything I want now. There is *no way* I will ever allow myself to go back to the old, 250-pound depressed guy I was before. I now realize how that 'old me' threatened my well-being, my health, and my life.'

"Tony went on, 'Whenever I'm asked how to do what I did, I tell people, 'If you want to put a smile on your face and feel great about yourself daily, then you have to make a change. You have to come and see and experience what life is like on this side, when you are lighter and healthier. And I'm proof you don't need to be athletic or experienced in the gym—anybody can do it. If I can do it, then so can you.'

"That's only half of Tony's story," Daniel remarks excitedly. "See, I continue to keep in touch with Tony, and I am even more happy to tell you that after two years, not only has Tony kept his promise to me and made his lifestyle changes permanent, but he also keeps looking better and better. Just look at his third photo there," Daniel says as he points to the far right photograph of Tony.

Daniel then stands up and slowly walks over to the white board, where he proceeds to pick up the blue marker he had used to write all the previous Lessons. He continues talking as he walks… "His workouts continue. He is still eating smarter. And he's found that life just keeps getting better and better. In fact, he recently told me he passed the SWAT team tests, something he would never have been able to do prior to his transformation. I am so inspired by Tony for keeping his promise and making his lifestyle changes a permanent part of his life.

"This is the next, sixth Lesson, Audrey," Daniel explains, as he starts writing on the white board…

LESSON #6: GET MOVING (AND STAY MOVING)

Consistency, when it comes to working out and losing weight, wins over time, every time.

"This is another reason I've gone wrong, Daniel," Audrey remarks, as Daniel goes back and underlines the word "consistency."

Audrey continues with her observation, "I've always started and stopped... started and stopped... pretty much *every* diet or exercise program I've attempted. If I didn't see results, right away within a week or two, I gave up. I *never* gave anything a chance. Worse, I never stayed consistent. I can now see why this is so important, especially when it comes to exercise and eating smart."

Audrey writes the sixth Lesson in her black book, as Daniel leans over and opens up one of the drawers in his desk.

THE WORKOUTS

Daniel pulls out a small pile of papers, neatly clipped together, and lays them out on the top of his desk.

"Here you go, Audrey, these are the same workouts I provided to Tony," Daniel explains as he slides the papers across the desk toward Audrey.

"I want you to have these," Daniel says as he points to the workout journal sheets. "Every workout is planned out for you... resistance training with weights and cardiovascular exercises... and don't worry, Audrey, explanations for all the exercises are included there too. If you don't understand how to do any of the exercises, you can also watch our video demonstrations, online, at our iSatori.com website. There, you'll find more of these workout journal sheets for you to download. And you'll also find lots of informative workout videos, explaining how to perform each of the exercises I recommend. It's important you follow proper form while you're training with weights and doing cardio exercises, so you don't injure yourself and you get the most from your workouts."

Audrey excitedly picks up the papers and fans through them.

HOMEWORK ASSIGNMENT

"Your homework assignment tonight is pretty simple, Audrey," Daniel says as he sits back down in his chair. "In fact, it's so easy, we're going to do it right now…"

Easy, huh? Audrey thinks to herself, eager to hear what her new homework assignment is.

"You have your iPhone with you, right?" Daniel asks.

"Yes, right here," Audrey replies as she pulls it out of her pocket.

"Here's what I want you to do… open up your calendar and make an appointment… a meeting request… *with yourself,*" Daniel says.

He goes on, "Pick a time you want to work out. I've noticed you go at lunchtime with Jocelyn, so maybe it's 1:00 until 2:00… Will that time work for you?"

Audrey nods her head in agreement, as she thumbs her phone's touchpad.

"Go ahead and set an appointment, with yourself, during that hour. Now, I want you to click 'reoccurrence' on that appointment, so it's in your calendar daily. You can let it expire at the end of the year, or set it for the next 90 days—that's up to you—but the further out, the better."

Audrey continues to type on her phone, setting the appointment, as she looks up and asks, "What should I put in the Subject Line and Location?"

"Well, how about 'Workout,' or 'My Transformation Workout'… and for the Location, just put the gym name or where you'll be doing your physical workouts. Just be sure to put a place, so it's acknowledged as such; otherwise, it won't seem real to you when it pops up on your reminders."

"Okay, I got it set. Five days a week, at lunchtime, I have my workout appointments set up in my calendar. Now, what about the weekends?"

Daniel smiles at her and then replies rhetorically, "Remember what we discussed—consistency wins over time, so it's important to be consistent with your workouts. Five days a week is good, but I'd really like you to work out six days a week, and rest on Sundays."

"Okay," Audrey replies with little hesitance, "Whatever works."

Daniel then notices, looking over at his clock, that it's past 6:00. He replies to Audrey, "It's getting late, you'd better get home to your kiddos—I'm sure they're ready to see their mom."

Audrey grabs her belongings and puts the workout journal sheets into her satchel bag, before putting on her raincoat, and rushing out the door.

As she drives away, she thinks about the description she had put into her calendar for her workouts. It reads: "My NEW Body in Progress!" She's a little nervous, yet also excited, to start her new workouts tomorrow...

Chapter Sixteen

WEEK SEVEN

Audrey sits at her desk, gazing almost aimlessly at her computer screen; all she can think about is her meeting with Daniel later this afternoon. She's feeling a little sad.

Today marks the seventh week, and with that, her last of the seven Lessons. She can't believe it. *Boy, time sure flies when you're in good company*, Audrey thinks to herself. Just then, she remembers that's Daniel's favorite saying. She must have picked it up from being around him so often over the last two months.

She can't help but think about all she's learned so far…

Lesson Number One: From Albert's story… she learned how to buddy-up and find a support system of people who truly care for her and help keep her accountable toward her goals.

Lesson Number Two: Unlocking her reasons, and finding her "why," is one of her favorites, not only because it involves Jocelyn's incredibly inspiring story but also because she was able to uncover the *real* reasons she wants to lose weight and transform her life.

Lesson Number Three: How to think big but start with small steps. Building on what she learned from Shari's story, called SMART goals, has helped her set specific direction toward what she *really* wants to achieve and create the action steps to get there.

Lesson Number Four: Learning to acknowledge, accept, and actually love her body type… like Kim Bowser did… and use a person's physique that is *built* more like hers has served as a constant source of inspiration.

Lesson Number Five: One of her favorite stories… Carla… taught her to stop looking outward for a "quick fix" and begin to look inward for a long-term, sustainable solution to losing weight and living a happier life.

Lesson Number Six: Despite her fears of walking into a gym, learning that exercise… moving her body… as Tony's story demonstrated… and doing practically *anything* that requires her to move and breathe is *more* beneficial to changing her entire body shape, helping her relieve stress and depression along with a whole host of other healthful benefits, than anything else.

IT REALLY IS SIMPLE

Audrey can't believe it. Over the past two months, she's learned *so much more* than she *thought* she knew over the last twenty or so years. Because, although she had tried practically every diet imaginable, for some reason, everything she is learning from Daniel's stories seems to be so surprisingly simple, yet so remarkably powerful.

Putting each new Lesson she's learned into practice, over the last seven weeks, Audrey can already see *and* feel the incredible differences they're making in her life. Her body is changing in ways she had never seen before. So is her outlook on life, which almost always seems more positive nowadays. So much so, even others around her are noticing too…

"Audrey. Audrey…? Audrey!" She hears in the distance, before she comes to and notices Daniel standing in her office doorway, trying to get her attention.

"You okay?" Daniel asks, after he feels like he has her attention, though Audrey hasn't said a word yet.

"Yeah… Yeah, I'm actually *better* than okay!" Audrey exclaims, as she looks up at Daniel and smiles.

"In fact, you know what, Daniel? …I'm not afraid to say, out loud, that I love my life, and I … I…" Audrey hesitates before she musters up the courage to finish and says to herself, under her breath, "I love my life, and I love my body." Then she says it out loud. "I *absolutely* love my life and my body! Things couldn't get much better, Daniel."

"Oh, but they will, Audrey. They will," Daniel responds with enthusiasm as he walks into her office and pulls up a chair in front of her desk. "Just like all the other success stories we have talked about, I can assure you, life will keep getting better and better. You have barely scratched the surface of how wonderful life really can be when you are lighter, healthier, and happier."

Audrey's excited to hear that from Daniel, but refrains from showing too much enthusiasm because she's at work. "I can't wait," she replies back to Daniel. "I can't wait to see how much better life really can get. I almost can't imagine, but I am beginning to believe it will.

"The funny thing is…" Audrey pauses.

"What's that? What's funny, Audrey?" Daniel senses Audrey is afraid to say what's on her mind.

"I guess it's not funny, but it just seems so strange to me that putting all of these Lessons into practice hasn't been too terribly difficult, yet their effects are so amazingly powerful. After *all* the years of struggling with my weight, and trying diet after diet, only to find them increasingly difficult to follow until I'd ultimately fail, so why is it that this all seems *so simple* now?"

"Good question, Audrey," Daniel's quick to reply, eager to get his words in. "Remember, it is *not* easy to do, but it *is* simple to follow. That is, as you've experienced firsthand, once you know the Lessons, and put them into practice, it's almost effortless, and the results, as you've also come to find out, are nothing short of miraculous."

Just as Daniel is finishing his sentence, Jocelyn, the office manager, comes up to the doorway and enthusiastically joins in the conversation, "And she looks *great*, doesn't she? Audrey keeps changing almost daily. Pretty soon, it'll be time for another complete wardrobe change—downsizing!" Jocelyn says with a wink.

"I need you. It's pretty urgent," Jocelyn then adds, as she points at Audrey.

Before Audrey can say anything, Daniel stands up to exit and pipes in, "Audrey, I was just coming to tell you I'll be a little late tonight, for our meeting… probably no more than 30 minutes. Is that okay with you?"

Audrey signals it's okay, as she grabs her phone and a pen, and gets up from her desk to be rapidly whisked away by Jocelyn.

THE LAST LESSON

Five-thirty at night. The sun has just started to set behind the tips of the mountains, so the office is beginning to darken. Audrey walks down the hall toward Daniel's office.

"Are you ready?" she asks softly, walking into Daniel's office.

"Yep! Perfect timing, Audrey," Daniel replies, with fervor. "Take a seat, please."

Before sitting, Audrey asks the obvious question, "What about the before and after transformation pictures…. Whose picture should I take down off the wall?"

"No one's," Daniel says as he stands up. "Not today. We won't need anyone's picture for today's lesson."

While a bit perplexed, Audrey has learned over the last few months that nothing really surprises her from Daniel. *I wonder what he's up to today,* she thinks to herself, but she isn't about to say anything.

"Today is a lesson about the *past, present, and future.*"

Daniel points to the chair next to Audrey, and says, "So, take a seat, please. Get comfortable. This is going to be a good one…"

Now Audrey is really puzzled but sits comfortably and waits for Daniel to begin sharing the final Lesson.

Daniel returns to his seat, leans back in his chair, crosses his legs, and looks out through the large windows, peering at the sun as it finishes setting over the Rocky Mountains. He clears his throat and begins telling a story...

POOR STEPHEN

"Audrey, I want to tell you about someone who is dear to me, named Stephen. Stephen grew up standing in line with his mother at their local food bank to get their monthly supply of powdered milk, bread, and cheese. They lived together in government subsidized apartments. Stephen didn't have much, but he was a happy kid. He had lots of friends and a mother who cared for him deeply. His mother later met a gentlemen—the apartment maintenance man, in fact—who would happily take on the parenting role as Stephen's soon-to-be Dad.

"Like most young boys, Stephen was pretty active as a kid, spending a lot of time playing sports and games outside with his neighborhood friends. But sadly, when it came to eating, he was misled. See, Stephen didn't have much in the way of 'role models' when it came to eating. That came from television commercials, surrounding fast-food restaurants, or whatever his friends were eating from their nearby 7-Eleven convenience store.

"He grew up eating sugary cereal for breakfast. Munching on onion chips and drinking a soda for lunch. And thinking his favorite fast-food Mexican restaurant was a gourmet dinner. He didn't know any better. And neither did his parents.

"Make no mistake about it, Stephen didn't eat this way because these foods were his only choices, rather because he actually thought they were perfectly acceptable. The television commercials had convinced him, and his parents, that a bowl of his favorite cereal was a *nutritious* way to start the day. He heard from his friends that chips were a *healthy* snack, and that a soda would give him much-needed *energy*.

"And his parents thought taking him to dinner for a fast-food taco would fill Stephen up with a hearty, wholesome meal. Little did he, or his parents, know but these types of foods were killing him. *Literally*."

Daniel pauses and turns to look directly at Audrey and sees she's caught up in the story with him. She nods at him as if urging him to continue.

"By the age of twelve, Stephen developed a stomach disorder. When he finally visited a doctor, it changed his life forever. The doctor informed him if he didn't change the way he ate, he would eventually end up in the hospital. Stephen was confused because he thought he was eating foods that were completely healthy. *Nothing*, however, could have been further from the truth.

"As you can imagine, hearing this kind of news scared Stephen tremendously. So much so, that on his own—with influence from his parents—he decided that very day to change the way he would eat."

"That's amazing," interrupts Audrey. "He must have been a very motivated kid."

Smiling, Daniel continues, "He soon bought some books and learned about how to read nutritional labels on foods, and he even did some research on ingredients to learn about everything he could to prevent him from getting sicker and winding up in the hospital. He learned the *right* foods from the *wrong* foods. He figured out what types of foods were hurting him and making him sick. And equally important, he discovered more about foods that would heal him and make him healthier.

"What's more, as Stephen went on to fundamentally change his eating habits, he found it completely changed the way he felt and, as he grew older, the way he looked. He eventually went on to add in working out with weights, and as a result, win a couple of local teenage and men's bodybuilding contests. Even more impressive, he become deeply involved in the nutrition business, and soon thereafter he wrote what would become a national best-selling book on Amazon.com that was about nutrition and supplements, called the *Sports Supplement Buyer's Guide*. To say Stephen changed his life for the better, after changing his eating habits, would be an understatement. That single event— his 'Satori' moment—changed his life *forever*. Today, Stephen teaches people how to completely transform their own physiques through eating smarter, living with a positive mindset, and working out.

"You see, Audrey," Daniel says as he again turns away from facing the window, to look directly at Audrey, "his parents didn't know."

Audrey looks back at Daniel with confusion and curiosity.

"Stephen's parents grew up without *really* understanding food. His parents fed Stephen what *they* ate growing up... what the television commercials persuaded them to... and frankly, whatever Stephen *wanted* to eat. They honestly didn't know they were hurting him. Their hearts were in the right place, as good parents, they just didn't know all that much about nutrition and frankly, no one at that time knew much about 'health food'.... Heck, it wasn't even a buzzword yet, like it is today."

Audrey's still a bit perplexed and wonders to herself, *where is Daniel going with this?*

"Stephen's inability to eat right was *not* his parent's fault. It was *not* his own fault. And, Audrey," Stephen clears his throat, as he stands up from the chair and walks around his desk, toward Audrey. With a serious look on his face, he begins to say, "The way you've eaten, up to this point in your life, is *not* your fault either," before he's interrupted.

"It's not my fault…" Audrey doesn't know if she's asking a question or making a statement to Daniel.

"That's right. *It's not your fault*, Audrey," Daniel continues.

"You didn't know any better. You tried *this* diet and *that* diet, where each one tried to persuade you which foods were right and which were wrong. But make no mistake, Audrey, you still didn't know any more than you did before and were likely more confused than ever. That's why you continually came up short and were unsuccessful in your efforts to lose weight and keep it off. *But that all changes today, Audrey.*"

Audrey still isn't sure where Daniel is taking this story…

"Everything changes today, Audrey," Daniel's voice begins to project louder as he becomes even more excited.

"Now, it's time to take *everything* you've learned over our last seven weeks together, and surrender to the fact that although it's not your fault… the way you ate and lived in the past… You *no longer* have any excuses. You now have *all* the tools you need to eat smarter and reach your dreams of becoming a lighter, healthier, more confident person."

Audrey's speechless, though she's nodding in agreement.

Daniel continues, "You have made the decision to make a permanent lifestyle change, and now it's time to put all the pieces together and *forever* change your life, for the better. Are you ready?"

Audrey is certainly ready but can't acknowledge or confirm Daniel's request, because she isn't quite sure what he is asking her to do.

"You see, Audrey, your Lesson today…" Daniel walks over to the white board and proclaims, "… your Lesson is that while you thought today was the end for you, and for our Lessons, today is in fact *merely the beginning of your journey…*"

Audrey has finally started to put the pieces of Daniel's story together, as she stands up and says excitedly, "*I get it.* I understand what you're saying. I know it's not my fault that I've eaten so poorly all these years. I understand I have the power to make these changes and eat smarter. And, more importantly, I have a responsibility to teach my children, and my entire family, to learn to eat better… live healthier… not just for me, but for them!

"Oh my gosh. *I get it,*" Audrey continues, getting more emotional, "I understand the bigger picture here. *This isn't just about me.* It's about my children. It's about my family. It's my responsibility to take *all* I've learned here with you, over the last two months, and help others I care about to walk on a new, healthier path. I have a personal responsibility to 'pay it forward,' now that I know the seven Lessons."

Daniel puts down the marker he was about to use and walks over to Audrey, putting out his arms and says, "I am so proud of you, Audrey. You got it. You figured out the biggest Lesson of all, all on your own."

Audrey is so caught up in the excitement that when she notices Daniel's arms extended, she lunges forward and gives him a quick hug. For a split moment, she feels awkward, but quickly lets that feeling go, as she realizes it was well-deserved and needed.

Audrey feels so relieved she has finally learned all the Lessons she needs to alter the direction of her life for the better and make what she knows will become permanent lifestyle changes that will completely transform her—physically *and* spiritually. She knows in that very moment, her life will *never* be the same again.

As they step back from each other, Audrey looks up at Daniel and says, "Thank you! Thank you for everything…"

Daniel interrupts, "Don't thank me. Thank yourself. You're the one who is doing this. This is your journey… and it's only the beginning…"

Daniel walks briskly over to his white board, picks up the blue marker again, and below the other six Lessons, he proceeds to write.

LESSON #7: MAKE A COMMITMENT

Accept that it's not my fault I didn't eat right and work out. Today is the day I have <u>committed</u> to make a permanent change and, through my very own successful transformation, will <u>help others</u> around me to walk in my footsteps.

Audrey tries to keep up, writing speedily in her black book, as Daniel blurts out, "You don't have to write the first part, about it not being your fault."

Finishing up and setting down her pen, Audrey responds, "Actually I think it's *all* important, so I went ahead and wrote it all down. If it weren't important, you wouldn't have written it down yourself," with a bit of a sly smile.

"I guess you're right, Audrey. I suppose it is important. I never thought of that," Daniel replies.

HOMEWORK ASSIGNMENT

Daniel sets the marker down and looks back at Audrey with a look of seriousness, "I'm going to give you your *final* homework assignment…"

Audrey interrupts, "Another homework assignment? I thought I was finished?"

"Not quite, Audrey," Daniel responds, amused, thinking she sounds like one of his daughters who's been given an extra assignment at the end of the school year. "We are not quite done… remember, it's the final Lesson, number seven, so we are not finished with our homework assignments until *after* this Lesson. However, this one, Audrey… this one is the most important one you will do. It also will likely be the *most* difficult one you've done yet."

That remark catches Audrey's attention. She quickly glances across the desk at Daniel and comments, "Toughest one yet?"

"Yes, the most difficult one yet," Daniel confirms. "Difficult for you, and difficult for your family. You're likely going to resist this one. But make no mistake, Audrey, this is the most important and incredibly powerful homework exercise you will do. I promise."

Audrey prepares to write down her final homework assignment, not knowing exactly what Daniel is going to say to her…

"Here's what I'd like you to do, when you go home tonight: **clean out your kitchen.**"

Thinking about her clean countertops at home, Audrey looks at Daniel like he's crazy.

Daniel continues, "Let me clarify. Now that you know good foods from bad foods, I want you to go through your refrigerator, your freezer, and your cupboards and throw away *everything* you know is not healthy or nutritious for you. This won't be easy. And if you need help trying to determine whether a food is good or not, please don't hesitate to call and ask me," Daniel says as he smiles.

"What about my kids' foods… you know, all the stuff they love, and the things I've bought for their lunches?" Audrey asks with genuine curiosity and a little concern.

"All of it," Daniel replies with sincere weight to his voice and goes on, "It *all* must go. Don't worry. We're going to replace it… And that's the second part of your homework assignment," Daniel concludes.

GET SHOPPING!

"The second part involves your children, though. *And this is very important.* Be sure to involve your children in the next part. That is, I want you to take your kids to the grocery store with you. I want you to all shop together as you buy you and your family their new, healthy, nutritious foods…. to replace the ones you just threw out."

"Oh, and don't forget," Daniel blurts out, "make sure you take home plenty of our Eat-Smart nutritional shakes and bars… you're going to need these, and I know you'll rely on them heavily, simply because you're so busy, and they're such an easy and healthy way to take the guesswork out of eating right."

Daniel continues, "While you're shopping and picking out foods, it's important you share with them what you're doing, why you're doing it, and how this change in the foods you will be eating is a new way of living—for you *and* them. Help them understand why certain foods are bad for them, and why others are healthy."

Daniel sits back down in his chair and proceeds to tell Audrey, "Trust me, I know how difficult this is going to be. But like we discussed, you now have a responsibility. You know better now. You have a responsibility not only to yourself but to your family and those you care so deeply about. You can teach them, too, how to eat smarter."

Audrey is energetically writing in her book, as Daniel goes on, "And remember, Audrey, it's our responsibility to give our children a chance… a chance at life that is better *and healthier* than ours. You know, our kids do what we do… say what we say… and, like it or not, eat what we eat. So it's time to use this opportunity to teach your children how to choose foods wisely. To choose ones that will help nourish their bodies, prevent them from gaining unnecessary body weight, and keep them healthy and free of diseases and sicknesses. Unlike what you've had to endure for most of your life, let's prevent our kids from having to struggle with their weight for the rest of their adult lives.

"Audrey," Daniel is the most serious she has seen him yet, "I need you to promise me you'll do this homework exercise. This is vitally important, and believe it or not, may very well be the one that determines whether you ultimately succeed in your life-changing transformation. Can you do this one *tonight*?"

"*Tonight?*" Audrey replies, with a subtle sigh, looking at her watch.

"Yes, you *must* do it tonight," Daniel retorts, "It's critical you not waste any time waiting to perform this exercise and, equally important, that you involve your children."

"Okay, I can do it. I've made it this far, and there is no turning back.

And, you're right, I feel compelled… I know I have a deep responsibility, now that I know how to teach my children the same. I will do it. I will do it tonight. *I promise!*"

Daniel can tell Audrey is being authentic and will do her homework assignment later that evening.

Startling both of them, Audrey's iPhone alarm goes off. She had set it for 7:00, so she wouldn't be too late picking up her boys from her mother's house after work since she knew she would be later than usual.

"I've got to get going, Daniel, but I promise, I will pick up my boys from Mom's and… she hesitates and then asks… "Would it be okay, though, if I took them shopping first, and then came home and threw out all the bad stuff?"

Daniel thinks about it for a moment, and replies, "Of course. That would work just fine. I never thought of doing it in that order, but I actually think it might work out better that way. Good luck, and Audrey, be sure to be honest with your kids as you go through the homework exercise. They'll appreciate it."

Audrey scurries to gather her things together and replies, "Actually, now that I think about it, I'm looking forward to doing this with my kids. I think it will not only be educational for them, but it will be fun and rewarding for me."

DANIEL'S CONFESSION

Audrey starts to turn and walk out when Daniel blurts out, "Audrey?"

She turns, and Daniel stands there staring back at her for a few seconds. It's starting to become an uncomfortable silence before he finally says, "Audrey, that little boy ..." he clears his throat, as he appears to be getting choked up, "That little boy... the story I told you tonight of the boy, Stephen... that was... that was me. That story was *my* story, as a young boy growing up." His eyes begin to glaze.

Audrey pauses for a split second, smiles, and says to Daniel, "I know." She quickly turns and walks out of Daniel's office.

Daniel stands in dead silence. He can't figure out how she already knew that story was about him. At the same time, he feels relieved, because he hasn't so openly and honestly shared his story with hardly anyone before.

Driving to her mother's house, Audrey begins rehearsing what she's going to say to her kids while they're shopping, picking out new foods that are likely foreign to them. She's anxious, a little scared, yet *really very* excited to begin the next step in her journey...

Chapter Seventeen

THE JOURNEY

Over the course of the next four months, Audrey experienced something she wasn't entirely ready for. To say it was a *deeply emotional journey* would be an understatement.

Audrey would struggle, within herself, about whether she would ultimately embrace or reject the Lessons she had learned, along with the new, positive lifestyle changes she was undergoing.

Thankfully, embrace would win out.

After failing at so many diets before, she had grown tired of losing confidence in herself and feeling hopeless about losing weight. Fortunately, she *fully* embraced the Lessons shared by her company's founder, Daniel, and found the strength and courage to follow her newfound habits.

Week after week drew her closer to her aspirations. Soon, she found herself growing more and more encouraged by the progress she was seeing in the mirror. What's more, everyone else around her also noticed the remarkable changes she was making in her body and attitude. From the other ladies in the office to her best friend, Tara, to her mom and sister, and most importantly, her husband and two boys. Everyone was *so deeply inspired by* the incredible improvements she made.

In time, Audrey would experience a truly inspirational transformation, physically *and* emotionally. But it didn't come easily.

During the months that followed her meetings with Daniel, she would experience sporadic periods of frustration, especially when she was around her "old" friends as they continued to try and persuade her to revert back to her "old" ways of eating.

Audrey also went through many bouts of disappointment, when she had "slip-ups" and got off course. But what she quickly realized was it was far easier to focus on her progress rather than on doing everything "just right" or perfectly.

On top of that, her time commitments of being a mother, wife, and having a full-time, demanding career pulled her attention in many different directions. Yet she came to appreciate that as long as her priorities were to take care of herself and improve her well-being, so she could better care for her family and others, she would feel less conflicted and more at ease with herself.

To make matters even better, in her moments of weakness, she continually found relief in knowing her answers were always only seven Lessons away. Over time, her new way of living simply became an automatic, almost effortless, way of thriving.

For the first time in her life, Audrey was genuinely happy with herself and felt confident in her physical appearance.

She *never* thought she could achieve the amount of weight loss she did… and she never thought in a million years she would ever consider what she was about to do.

Chapter Eighteen

THE TRANSFORMATION

One year later, Audrey had lost an *incredible* 113 pounds.

She went from a weighty 260 pounds down to a beautiful and healthy 147 pounds.

Her transformation was remarkable.

In fact, on more than one occasion, people who hadn't seen her in over a year honestly couldn't believe she was the same person. They even remarked as such. But it *was* Audrey.

The weight Audrey lost resulted in her now having a completely different outlook on life. The lenses through which she now saw her life were so much more positive… so much happier… and so much more confident.

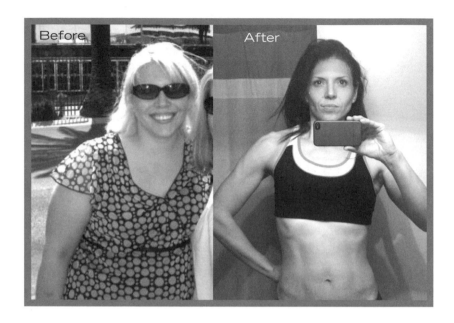

Before

After

Simply put, the physical changes Audrey made on the outside were a mere reflection of the changes she made on the inside.

She was a better role model and mother to her kids.

She was a better wife and friend to her husband, Joe.

She was a happier person to be around with her friends and sister.

She was more confident about her body when she went to the gym to work out, and it showed.

She was more self-assured and assertive at her job and started making significant advancements in her career.

She was more poised and secure in her self-image, and as a result, she carried herself with so much more pride, though she stayed grounded in the humility of always remembering her struggles as a child, and where she had started this journey.

It was noticeable to *everyone* around her that her transformation had a positive effect on literally *all* other parts of her life!

She felt content and complete, though she knew—deep down—this was only the beginning.

A wonderful beginning to a *brand new* chapter in her life. She was more excited than ever before.

SURPRISE

Audrey surprised herself—and everyone else around her—when one day she announced she would enter a local "figure" fitness contest.

Before now, this was so far out of her league, she would never have had the confidence to step on a stage and let others judge her physical appearance, but now the idea intrigued her.

She wanted to prove to herself she could do it. She could set a new goal and carry through with it.

This would be a remarkable and most memorable moment in her life. It would be fun. It would be an "exclamation point" on her transformation. And it would be rewarding!

Over the coming months, as she prepared for her competition, Audrey found herself in a peculiar place. That is, she discovered that along her journey, as other people witnessed her weight-loss transformation firsthand, they sought her out for help.

She was humbled by people coming to her to seek her advice on nutrition, working out, and losing weight. Yet she was happy to share her story and the Lessons she had learned from Daniel.

THE JOYS OF SUCCESS

Why did Audrey succeed at her weight-loss transformation, while so many other dieters fail?

Some would say she is an extraordinary woman. While that *is* true, I am not sure that's all there is to it. While Audrey certainly possesses a great number of amazing personal qualities, in many ways, she is quite an ordinary woman. She has a full-time job, family responsibilities, and children to attend to. She also has her fair share of setbacks and problems, just like anyone else. So I would argue it was her *courage* to make a firm decision to embrace change; her *willingness* to accept new lifestyle habits; combined with her inner *strength* to actually act on them in a consistent and meaningful manner. This, in totality, helped her create a remarkably inspiring transformation.

What she found interesting and somewhat surprising was that, along her journey, she became a source of inspiration to others around her.

A day doesn't go by when someone close to her doesn't make a comment about her transformation progress, and then ask her how they could do the same.

Soon, Audrey found herself assisting those who sought out her help, to learn how they too could walk in her footsteps. She provided them the spark they needed to make a decision to change. She found herself sharing the very same Lessons Daniel had taught her. She told the same stories he did. She provided the plan and path they needed to achieve their dreams of a new body and improved health. She became their greatest supporter and a "success coach"—something she never could have imagined before today.

FINDING HOPE

The good news about Audrey's story is there is hope for us too. Because *we too* can become incredibly inspiring transformational success stories if we surrender to the fact that "diets" will *always* fail us. (Let's face it: they flat out suck!)

Instead, if we embrace the fact that weight-loss success is not so much a function of willpower or deprivation, but rather of our decision to change and our commitment to see our dreams become a reality.

But there is the potential for bad news here too. We can stay the same in our habits, or follow the next fad diet that comes along, or worse, we can close this book, tuck it away on the bookshelf—only to let it collect dust—and never take any action whatsoever on the Lessons learned here.

The choice is yours to make.

Promise me, though, you won't do the latter. Please.

Instead, let's start our journey together, right now, by turning the page and embracing the next step by learning exactly how Audrey put all the pieces together... see how she lives her life now by exploring "a day in the life of Audrey"... and learn how you can easily put each Lesson learned into practice in your own life...

THE MODEL

Chapter Nineteen

THE MODEL

Putting All the *Lessons* Together and Into Practice

As simple as it is to undergo a transformation and build a better body, make no mistake, *it is not easy*. The good news, though, it is not all that complicated. In truth, keeping it simple is critical.

Whether you are 81 or 21 years old, or whether you are a busy executive, or a working mother, or if you are a full-time student or a truck driver, if you put into practice the Seven Lessons, I am *absolutely, positively* certain you too can make a *truly* impressive, life-changing transformation.

How do I know this?

From the thousands upon thousands of people I have helped over the past 20 years both personally and through my books, articles, and online resources, that's how. They have inspired me, and more importantly, taught me that once these Lessons are put into practice, remarkable things will begin to happen. It is like living in the dark and suddenly finding the light switch.

Unfortunately, this is where, for most people, it is quite common to struggle with *how* to go about making it happen. That is, how to put everything together and put the *Lessons* into practice—in *your own* life. If you feel this way, you are not alone. In fact, it is *exactly* how Audrey felt, even though she had learned all the Lessons she needed to create change after her weekly meetings with Daniel.

BABY STEPS

The first step is to *never, ever* give up hope that you *can* create change in your life. As long as there is a tomorrow, this new day presents you with another opportunity to change.

The second step is to embrace the idea that, unlike anything else you may have tried before, a life-changing transformation requires an extraordinary amount of commitment, courage, and consistency.

The third, and most important step, is to go back and review the *Lessons*—let each one resonate with you, do the "homework assignments" yourself, and begin to put them into practice daily. Or, if you prefer to take it a little slower, put them into practice on a weekly basis. Whatever works, *for you.*

The rest of this book is designed to provide a clear, concise, and practical path to putting the *Lessons* into practice, in your own life, to transform your physique and your life.

PUTTING THE PLAN INTO ACTION

Most people spend a considerable amount of time and energy, over many countless attempts, following weight-loss strategies that inevitably fail. Usually trying things like crazy fad diets, frozen pre-portioned foods, weight-loss clinics, or other quick-fix gimmicks. This is unnecessary. It is not smart. What is smart, however, is practicing a small set of principles over a long period of time.

Recall, at the beginning of this book, I shared that small changes can have a big, and oftentimes, dramatic effect. This is true, so long as they are done with consistency *and* purpose.

A year after Audrey's transformation, she looks even better than she ever has. To her dismay, however, it took longer for Audrey to *see* herself the way others saw her. She had worked hard to change her physical appearance, and successfully did so over time, yet she struggled to see herself as the new, thinner, lighter, more attractive person she had become on the outside. This is a natural occurrence in transformations. Thankfully, in time, she began to feel more comfortable with her new appearance, and she finally began to see herself as others did.

And so to provide you with a perfect example of living out the *Lessons* Audrey experienced and lived day in and day out, it is best to show you, firsthand, exactly what a typical day for Audrey looks like and how she puts each one into practice. (Read this section carefully, please, because she is a great example of how you can put them into practice in your life, too!)

Chapter Twenty

A DAY IN THE LIFE OF AUDREY

AS TOLD BY HER

First, I can't overstate the importance of planning. Before I even consider anything else, I always, always make sure I have my entire day planned out. For me, there could be nothing more integral to my success. In fact, whenever I don't plan my days, I notice everything feels "out of control" the next day. And it usually is.

That's why I always take about 15 to 20 minutes each night, before I go to bed, and look over my next day's workout and ensure it's scheduled in my calendar, prepare my meals to take to work, write out my most important to-dos, and as corny as it sounds, even pick out my clothes to wear. I can't tell you how much time this nightly ritual saves me, and how much more organized I feel the next day. If you're already good at planning, then you'll certainly agree. If not, then I'd encourage you to start tomorrow and adopt this terrific habit.

So now let's take a closer look at how I incorporate the *Lessons* you just learned and allow me to share with you exactly how I apply them in my life.

Luckily, a great deal of the planning "work" for the exercise routines has already been done for you, by Daniel, in the Workout Program he's put together (and you can download the worksheets at iSatori.com in the workout section). In there, just as he did for me, Daniel laid out the days you should exercise. Pointed out exactly which body parts to work out. He even planned the exact number of sets, reps, and time to rest for each workout. On top of that, he included a full week of sample meals—from breakfast to lunch to snacks to nighttime meals and even desserts—so you can *easily* put together your daily eating plan.

By the way, I'm not saying these are the only ways to exercise and eat, but they are what I used, and they worked marvelously well for me and the thousands of other successful transformations Daniel has shared them with. And, I am certain, with little modification, they can work just as well for you too.

Believe me, when you look at how much of the guesswork Daniel has taken out of losing weight and transforming your physical appearance, and how carefully designed these workout programs are, it doesn't get much simpler than this. In fact, I wish someone had shown me a program like this when I first started out, when I was younger and struggling with my weight. It would have saved me years and years of failure and disappointment.

Anyway, let's get back to putting the *Lessons* into practice... and by way of example, take an in-depth look at how I put everything together: On page 199, you'll see an example of how I fill out the exercise portions of the program. This page is appropriately called "Sample Workout Sheet."

Now, because Daniel has already laid out the body parts to train, exercises, sets, reps, and rest times, there's only one thing left for you to plan—the "goal" weights and times. Although it's easy to do, you should take your time and carefully examine your past workouts and the weights you used and duration of the workouts to determine which weights and times you should write down for your next workout.

If you haven't worked out before, please don't be afraid. Daniel has also provided full video examples of each workout, exercise lift, and detailed explanations. You can find these, too, on iSatori.com. (I refer back to these videos all the time, whenever I get puzzled by an exercise or new lift I haven't done before; and they're even fun to watch for a refresher from time to time.)

You won't find this in my examples here, but because I'm always trying to push myself, I usually tack on about five to ten percent more weight and slightly increase the intensity of my cardio exercise about every couple of weeks. This way, I'm sure to keep my progress coming along. Plus, it's a great way to set your sights a little higher to really help push yourself.

Once I've planned my Workout Sheet for the next day, I move on to my nutrition plan. Here is where I'll outline exactly what I plan to eat. From the first to the last meal, including any supplements, and how much water I plan to drink. I don't like to leave anything to chance, and as a result, I usually stay right on course each day. Honestly, I've found the closer I follow my plan, the faster I reach my goals. *There are really no two ways about it.*

I've provided a blank Daily Nutritional Planning Sheet on page 202 (you can download and make copies of the same blank Daily Nutritional Planning Sheet at iSatori.com under the *Diets Suck!* tab), and use it to plan and write out your meals each day. Later in this chapter, you may notice my total calories are somewhat higher than the examples provided on iSatori.com. That's because I weigh around 146 pounds, I'm five foot ten, which is pretty tall for a woman, and I'm training pretty intensely these days, and the examples I've provided are for a 150-pound person who is sedentary. You might weigh more or less than this, or exercise more or less than I do, so you'll need to calculate your daily protein needs for your desired weight-loss goal.

Once you do that, it's pretty easy to plan your meals. From there, you can pick and choose which food choices most closely match your preferences for particular foods and then adjust them, based on portion sizes, to meet your protein needs. Now that I've written out the meals I plan to eat the following day, I'm about 50% done with my planning.

Next, I prepare the meals I am going to eat. I do this at the same time I am preparing my kids' lunches. It makes it easier for me. Since tomorrow is going to be a busy day for me (and I have a late luncheon meeting), I plan on eating two whole-food meals and having two meal-replacement protein shakes during the working day. Knowing that, I'll need to make the meals in advance. Again, so I leave nothing to chance.

To make my foods for the next day, I prepare a chicken breast with a lettuce and tomato salad, steamed brown rice, which I put in a Tupperware bowl, and I grab an apple (Gala are my favorite), a large bottled water with lots of ice, and all of my nutritional supplements. I put everything in my shoulder bag and keep it in the refrigerator to take to work with me the next day. I always double-check my supplement case to make sure I've got enough supplements to last me the entire day.

Since I'm going to have two protein nutrition shakes tomorrow, I'm sure to pack two Blender Bottles, each with a scoop of Eat-Smart shake mix inside them. This way, all I have to do is add water and some ice cubes, shake it up, and I have a healthy "meal" in less than one minute. I can't tell you how grateful I am for the Eat-Smart nutrition shakes. They honestly taste like a milkshake, keep me full for hours, and really take the time and guesswork out of eating right. And, thankfully, they don't bloat me or give me gas, like most protein shakes tend to do.

(If you don't have a Blender Bottle, I'd encourage you to get one. They are pretty inexpensive and very convenient to use for carrying and mixing your protein shakes. You can buy one online at iSatori.com, Bodybuilding.com, or at your local GNC store.)

Because I like to eat breakfast with my two boys, yet we seem to always be in a rush in the mornings, I put out on the counter most of our breakfast foods, like oatmeal, and condiments like stevia sweetener. And since I usually drink about two meal-replacement protein shakes every day, I keep a spare container of Eat-Smart at the office, so I don't need to lug it back and forth, from my home to work, and more importantly, so I never leave myself without a healthy "back-up" meal, just in case I don't have enough food or forget to bring my Blender Bottles filled with Eat-Smart powder.

Now that I've written out my goal weights and times for my next workout; written out and prepared the meals I plan to eat tomorrow; made sure I've got the nutritional supplements I need to use, the final thing I do is prepare my clothes. Since I work out at lunchtime, during the workday, I make sure I have packed in my gym bag a comfortable T-shirt, pair of spandex or shorts, socks, sports bra, and underwear, and my tennis shoes. Last, I make sure I've got my iPhone. (iTunes is my favorite digital headphone music system. To be honest, I couldn't exercise without this: it genuinely helps give me energy and keeps my intensity up while working out and just gives me so much more motivation to push myself.)

After this, I'm off to bed. It's usually around 10:00 or 10:30 p.m. The next morning, *just like I do every day,* I wake up at 5:00 a.m. Without hesitation, before getting dressed, I head for the kitchen and pour a large glass of water. There's nothing more refreshing, and important, than a tall glass of water first thing in the morning. Especially considering your body hasn't had any food or liquids for about seven or eight hours. A year ago I would have made a cup of coffee at this point—before doing anything else—to help "get me going" and wake me up. But I don't feel this way any longer.

I head back upstairs to my kids' bedrooms to wake them before showering and getting myself dressed for the day. Once my boys are dressed and ready to go, we head back downstairs and all have breakfast together. This is one of my favorite parts of the day. I make them apple sauce, yogurt, or eggs and toast or their absolute favorite, if we have time, "protein pancakes"; and I usually make a small bowl of oatmeal with Eat-Smart for myself. If we are really rushed for time, I will make myself an Eat-Smart meal-replacement nutrition shake, and I'll even pour some for the kids (they love it), or I'll grab them an Eat-Smart nutrition bar to eat in the car on the way to school.

Either way, I make sure to never, ever miss out on eating breakfast— for me or my boys. It's frankly the *most important* meal of the day. Daniel once showed me some peer-reviewed scientific studies that showed people who ate breakfast, and didn't skip it regularly, were four times *less* likely to be overweight. *Four times.* This was pretty convincing for me.

Once everyone is finished with breakfast, we brush our teeth, gather our things, including our lunch sacks, and head out of the house for the day.

After I drop off my boys at school, I usually arrive at the office a few minutes before 8:00 a.m. By the time I get everything put away in the refrigerator and get settled at my desk, it's only a few more minutes before the office really starts buzzing… the phone starts ringing, and the emails start piling up.

I take a deep breath, look over my daily to-dos, review my calendar for the appointments I have that day (including my lunch appointment to work out!), and then I pause to look at the picture of my kids, and the before and after pictures of myself, where I say out loud: "*I love my body. I love my family. I love my life!*" I say this three times, with complete sincerity and joy, before I officially get started on my workday. This morning ritual makes me feel *so good* inside and confident about myself.

I look at my clock on the computer, and it says 10:00 a.m. That means it's time to eat again. See, as I learned from Daniel, eating smart… that is, eating small, frequent meals throughout the day, versus depriving myself through crazy diets, which I used to do, or overeating once or twice a day, helps keep me well nourished, my energy is stable throughout the day, and my body is actually burning more body fat than it stores.

It's been about three hours since I ate breakfast, and when I glance over my nutrition plan for the day, I have "chicken, salad, brown rice, and half an apple" written down. So, I head back to the kitchen to grab it out of the refrigerator. I also make sure to pour a tall glass of iced water.

After I have my meal together, I sit down with whoever else might be in the kitchen and strike up a conversation, which could either be work-related or personal. I find this is a great time to *really* get to know the others I work with, even deeper. It makes it feel much more like a family than a workplace. That's what I love *most* about working at iSatori—everyone feels like they are family to me.

Time flies at work, and before I know it, the appointment for me to work out pops up on my Outlook calendar on the computer around 12:45 p.m. It's time to go to the gym and exercise. It's time to take care of myself, as I happily see it.

I get butterflies pretty much every time this reminder comes up. I know it sounds silly, but it's just the way I feel when I get excited. And for some strange reason, working out and knowing I'm taking care of myself and improving my health and physical appearance gets me anxious and even a little giddy—in a good way. What's more, because I go to the gym with a few of my friends in the office, I get excited to work out with them and help share with them what I have learned so far. *It's really fun.*

I know I have to drive to the gym and complete my workout, within an hour, so I rush off to the ladies' washroom to change into my workout clothes. (We have a shower and changing room, so it's really convenient.) I have everything with me, and ready, so it takes me only a few minutes. Afterward, I walk by the others' desks and signal it's time to go work out, and we all carpool together to the 24-Hour Fitness near the office. It's only a couple of minutes away, so we listen to music on the ride over and talk about what we will be working that day.

Since they all look to me for guidance, I simply pull out my Workout Planner and show them what we will be doing that day in the gym. It's easier for them this way and makes it more purposeful for me. Having this support system also keeps me, and them, more accountable to our workouts. It's difficult to miss a workout when you know there are others counting on you. Plus, we have all been doing this now for almost a year, so it's a daily ritual for us. We really couldn't imagine our day *any* other way.

When we arrive at the gym, we are all ready to go. We have about 45 minutes to work out, so we don't waste any time and get right to it. After getting my iPhone ear-bud headphones plugged in with my favorite music, I'm ready to start training. Today we are going to work out our upper bodies, which includes chest, back, shoulders, biceps, and triceps. We are going to follow the "5-4-3-2-1 workout system" Daniel showed me awhile back, and I've followed ever since.

We start by picking out the four exercises we will do today for the body parts being trained. We chose dumbbell bench press for chest; lat pull downs for back; seated dumbbell side lateral raises for shoulders; preacher curl machine for biceps; and bar dips for triceps. (See the "Training" section at iSatori.com for a detailed explanation and demonstration videos for all the exercises in this program.) There are five of us, so each person is assigned to a workout station. This way, we can each perform the exercise we start at, and then rotate to the next exercise. We simply follow this order, each of us rotating from one exercise to the next, without resting in-between sets, until we have completed one full cycle of all five body part exercises.

I start the chest workout with flat dumbbell bench presses. I prefer dumbbells to barbells when doing bench press because it doesn't cause any pain in my shoulders, like a barbell does. To get my muscles warmed up and get the blood flowing in my body, I start by using 10-pound dumbbells for a "warm-up" set of 15 to 20 repetitions—using a moderate level of intensity. This set is not scheduled on my workout planning sheet, but I feel it's important to do.

Without resting, I walk over to the next exercise—the lat pull down. This is a seated exercise with a straight overhanging bar. I use 40 pounds on the machine and again perform another warm-up set of 15 to 20 repetitions. The next exercise is for shoulders. For this we've chosen side lateral raises with dumbbells. I grab the five-pound dumbbells and take a seat on a flat bench, and perform the exercise, doing at least 15 to 20 warm-up repetitions. By now, I am starting to breathe a little harder and can feel my body's intensity meter move up. I set the dumbbells back onto the rack and walk over to our next exercise—preacher curls for biceps (the front muscle on the arm). It's a machine, so I plug the pin on the weight stack into the 25-pound marker and do my first warm-up set of 15 to 20 repetitions. Finally, on the last exercise in our workout rotation, I will do another 15 to 20 repetitions of bar dips for my triceps (the back of the arm).

Once I'm finished with the last exercise, that completes one full rotation of our workout program. This is the first *giant set* as I call them.

At this time, we all take a breather for a short while—actually 60 seconds to be precise. We watch the clock closely. We don't spend time chatting with each other, instead we get a drink of water, stretch, or focus on our breathing. Afterward, we start the same rotations all over again. We do this four more times. Each time we go through the rotation, however, we progressively increase the weights used and decrease the number of repetitions (normally starting from 20 and moving down to 12, 10, 8, and again 8 repetitions). This way, we can push ourselves to get stronger and more shapely muscles by improving our weight and varying our repetitions. This was another important fact Daniel shared with me, when he showed me a pile of scientific studies explaining the need to change up training variables, like weight, repetition, and even the order in which you perform the exercises. This completes the 5-4-3-2-1 workout system— five completed giant sets. This took us about 23 minutes.

Now, we each pick our favorite cardiovascular exercise machine, where we will finish out our workout. I usually pick the one we all affectionately call "Big Bertha." It's a stair-stepper. I like to switch it up, though, and will use either the Spinning stationary bike or the Elliptical. Once I get started, I set the timer for 20 minutes and use a pretty high intensity level. Again, Daniel shared with me countless additional scientific studies that showed doing cardiovascular exercise for shorter, more intense durations was actually more beneficial for burning excess calories and body fat than low intensity for longer periods of time. By the time I have completed my 20 minutes, I am winded and barely able to carry on a conversation.

Now, we're done.

Today's weight-training and cardiovascular workout took approximately 43 minutes. Two minutes under my goal of 45 minutes. By this time, all of us, especially me, are sweating, and our hearts are racing. But, you know, this is where I feel *the most* alive. After sitting all morning at a desk, the truth is, *nothing* feels better to me than getting in the gym and feeling alive by working out. I feel *so* invigorated when I'm done.

We gather our belongings and head back to the office, where we shower and get our "work" clothes back on. Well, not always. The funny thing is, because we work at a health and fitness company, it's not uncommon for us not to change back into our regular clothes but instead keep our workout clothes on. It's a neat part of our company's culture. Another reason I *love it* there so much!

I'm often asked why I work out with weights, and since I'm a woman, whether I'm afraid of getting too muscular. Honestly, I used to be afraid of the same thing. Interestingly, though, after talking with Daniel, and doing my own research, I discovered working out with weights will not make me muscular or bulky. For starters, as a woman, I don't have enough of the hormone called testosterone in my body, so it's virtually impossible to put on muscle, fast.

Aside from that, training with weights and sculpting lean body mass is actually the *only* (let me repeat that for emphasis), the *only* way to reshape your body. It's the only way to trade in ugly, unsightly body fat for lean, sexy, curvy muscle. What's more, muscle mass is "metabolically active," meaning just by having more of it, it causes your body to naturally burn more body fat. And, let's not forget, there are many, many health benefits to weight training, like improving bone density (which is very important for men, but especially women), and increasing energy levels by elevating your body's chemicals in the brain that make you feel happy and joyful.

That's why several scientific studies have shown that exercise, especially training with weights, can alleviate depression and suppress anxiety. It's easy to see why working out is so essential to living a happy, healthy life, and the only way to truly transform your physical appearance.

Whenever I work out, I push myself as hard as I can, *without sacrificing my form,* until I am completely exhausted and can't budge the weights any longer. Between each set, I pay close attention to the amount of time I rest and am careful not to exceed the time listed on my workout sheet. Not only does this help keep the intensity of my workout peaked, but it also ensures I'll get my workouts done in a timely manner—*in well under an hour.* To keep better track of time, I wear a wristwatch that has a built-in timer and heart-rate monitor. I suggest you get one or something similar to keep track of your rest periods. I can't stress how important this is to maximizing your intensity by keeping track of your time.

I also use my rest periods to write down both my "actual" weights used and my "actual" number of reps performed. **This is very important to journal,** so when you're planning the next workout, you can reference the weights you used and time you spent in the gym, and include them in your "goal" weights and times. (You can increase, or decrease them, depending on whether you reached or exceeded your goals.)

Remember, when you do your workouts, you might use less or more weight than I do. That doesn't really matter. What matters most is you keep a constant record of the actual weights and reps you did and pay close attention to the time you rest between sets. This way, you're sure to keep your intensity levels up and make the most of your time spent in the gym. I also use this time to jot down a few notes about the workout. For instance, today I repeatedly noticed how good my arms were looking. These were always a "problem area" for me, and there's some loose skin and fat on the backs of my arms, but today they looked noticeably better, and I'm pretty excited about it, so I jotted that down on my workout journal sheet.

I got a great, intense workout, and everyone did a terrific job of keeping pace. In fact, I'll need to make a note for the next time we train upper body that I should increase the weights used since everything felt a little "lighter" today. *This is all very important information to record.* And this is it for the exercise portion of my day.

Following the 5-4-3-2-1 workout system means I train with weights three days a week, on Mondays, Wednesdays, and Fridays, along with cardiovascular exercise. (See The Workouts section for your full 12-week calendar workout schedule on page 203.) When I made my transformation, **I followed this calendar to the letter.** In fact, like I said earlier, the closer I follow my plan, the faster I see results, and the greater my progress. On the alternate days—Tuesdays, Thursdays, and Saturdays—we perform additional cardiovascular exercise. This type of exercise is not only good for improving the condition and strength of your heart, but it also works wonders to help your body become much more efficient at burning off unwanted body fat.

For our cardiovascular exercise days, normally the same ladies and I walk over to the nearby county fairgrounds and run intervals up and down the stadium stairs. We do this by running for three minutes and then walking for one minute. We alternate like this for a total of 30 to 40 minutes. It's pretty exhausting, but again, like going to the gym and weight training, when you are done with cardiovascular exercise, you feel so much better about yourself and so alive. As long as the weather is nice outside, we will go and run the stairs. I find this is more enjoyable than running on a treadmill or using the stair stepper at the gym.

But, if weather doesn't permit, we will certainly make our way to the gym for our cardio exercise. Interestingly, though, we have found a way to make it more fun at the gym than the usual by alternating cardio machines, every five to seven minutes, in the same rotational pattern we do with our weights. That is, we switch and use five different cardio machines. We have found this routine makes doing cardio more fun and really makes the time go by so much faster. Before we know it, we're finished, and it's time to go.

The workouts are pretty simple. Maybe not easy to do, but certainly simple to follow, wouldn't you agree? And best of all, they take no more than one hour a day. When you put it into perspective, that's only three and half percent of your time during the week. That doesn't seem like much time to commit to something that will dramatically improve your health and completely change your physique! Remember, it's the small changes, over time, that have dramatically powerful effects. This is one of them.

By the time I walk back into my office, my mind is refreshed, and I'm ready to take on the rest of the day's challenges.

Now, it's just after 2:00 and time to eat. But not just any meal will do. Because I just worked out, my body is primed for quality nutrients to help it recover and renew my energy. As Daniel taught me, this is where I want to pay careful attention to what I put into my body. With this meal, we want to feed our muscles and starve our fat. *This time is called our "open window."* Our bodies will literally soak up anything we feed them during this time. That's why it's critical to feed ourselves quality protein and carbohydrates and other important nutrients. I do this by making an Eat-Smart meal-replacement protein shake.

This shake has the highest quality proteins to help my muscles recover from the strenuous exercises; it contains healthy carbohydrates from oats to help support healthy cholesterol levels and keep me feeling fuller for longer. It also has added fiber, to keep the digestive track more regular, and it contains probiotics for healthy, "good bacteria" in the gut. It also has enzymes to help assimilate the protein better, so you won't have any gas or bloating.

I simply put 12 ounces of water in the blender and add three or four ice cubes and one rounded scoop of my Eat-Smart Double Vanilla Ice Cream flavor. (This is my favorite flavor, by the way—it tastes like melted ice cream on the bottom of the bowl.) Then, because I want to add a little more flavor and for added healthy carbohydrates, I add about one-half cup of frozen strawberries. I blend this on high for about 45 seconds. The strawberries give the shake a fruity taste—*a lot like* one of those frozen tropical fruit smoothies you get while on vacation in Mexico.

Now, in less than one minute, I've got a chilled, thick, rich shake with the nutrition my body is craving, including whey protein, probiotics, and hunger-satisfying fiber. I've now provided myself with the perfect amount of carbohydrates and protein, and important vitamins and minerals. **It's shortly after 2:00 by now**, and this "smart meal" will keep me satisfied for another two to three hours, at least.

Keep in mind, all throughout the day, and in between my meals, I'm continually drinking from a large water bottle I keep at my desk. It is really important to stay hydrated, especially since I just trained as well and lost a great deal of water through perspiration.

At 4:00 in the afternoon, I'm ready for my fourth meal of the day. I don't have much time to spare, so I make this meal quick and simple. In fact, I call this meal my "fast-snack." It's really nothing more than a small cup of Greek yogurt (sugar free), and I sprinkle on and mix in some Muesli grains cereal. This is a terrific, very healthy snack too. Daniel showed me this one day while we were taking a break together in the kitchen, and I've loved it ever since. I keep a large container of fresh, plain Greek yogurt in the office refrigerator, so it's always available. I also cut up the Gala apple I brought with me into small slices. Next, I pour a tall glass of ice water. And that's it—my fourth meal. *Really not all that complicated, is it?*

This meal, though it may seem strangely timed at around 4:00 is actually like a mid-day "break" to me. It's a time to close my door and sit at my desk for a few minutes while I eat by myself and reflect upon the day. I use this time to think about all I've accomplished during the day. It's a pretty fast-paced company, so it's easy to forget all you've done. More importantly, I use this time to review my goals, both personally and professionally. I know it sounds corny, but I must confess, I have found the more often I do this "exercise," the more aware it makes me of the goals I've set for myself and the closer I feel I've come to achieving them.

While reflecting, I think about the reasons I am working so hard at the office, in order to advance my profession and to take good care of my family; and I think about the reasons I continue to work out so hard at the gym and eat so well during the days. Whereas before, my motivation was because I didn't want to look like my "before" picture, now it is because I have become a role model to my children, sister, and mom, who are all eating smarter and living more active lives. And because I have become a source of inspiration and guidance to the other women in the office, and they are counting on me to help them.

Honestly, a year ago if you asked me if I could have seen myself in the position I'm in today, I wouldn't have guessed I would be where I am. Though my reasons have changed, I am still as motivated as ever before to continue to look and feel better about myself and probably more so now than ever before.

I usually leave the office around 6:00 in order to pick up my boys from my mother's. Tonight, I promised them we would go out to dinner, since there wasn't any school today, and it was mommy's special celebration—after losing 100 pounds. After picking up my two boys and chatting with my mother for a few minutes, we head to our favorite restaurant around 7:00. This will be my fifth meal of the day, and since we are eating out, I won't need to prepare anything at home for dinner.

We head to dinner at one of our favorite nearby restaurants, Olive Garden. We like this place because it's very family-friendly, and they have lots of good dishes to choose from. And my kids like that you can eat all the salad you want. They absolutely love salad. We also like this specific Olive Garden, near our house, because the servers, managers, and cooks know us very well. (Keep this in mind the next time you go out to eat. Try to choose places where you can visit regularly and employees can become familiar with *your* eating habits.) I find this helps. A lot. They don't look at me like I'm crazy when I ask for "dressings on the side" or an "added grilled chicken breast," or "make that without butter please." This is important because I don't want to miss out on being able to socialize and have any meal at a restaurant, whether it's breakfast, lunch, or dinner, with family or friends. It's good to become familiar with restaurants that will happily accommodate your "healthy" eating requests. If they don't, then I usually won't eat there any longer.

Today, just like most days when I visit Olive Garden, I order angel hair pasta, no butter or cream sauce, with olive oil, a grilled chicken breast, and sun-dried tomatoes. It's a perfect combination of complex carbohydrates, good quality proteins, and even essential fats (from the olive oil). With dinner, I drink a glass of iced tea with a packet of Splenda sweetener in it.

I use this opportunity to order healthier meals for my kids, too, instead of deep-fried foods or whatever they serve on the "children's menu." I order them grilled chicken, diced into small cubes, and regular spaghetti pasta, with marinara sauce. Their choice of drinks are milk (2%), water, or tea. No sodas. It did take a few months of eating this way, but with a little persistence, and sharing with them how unhealthy certain foods are, and how we're respecting their bodies and health, they came around slowly. Now, they don't mind at all. In fact, they don't like the other foods they used to order.

We all have a good time at dinner, talking about our day and the fun stuff we did. We finish up and head home so my kids can get ready for bed, and I can prepare myself for another productive day.

After I get the boys off to sleep, at around 8:30 p.m., I usually clean up a bit around the house, throw in a load of laundry, and then sit down in bed and read one of my many books. This is oftentimes my most cherished time. It's quiet, and I'm relaxed and in my own world. *It feels good.*

At about 9:30 p.m., I find myself craving something sweet or a desire for chocolate, so I head for the kitchen to make an Eat-Smart pudding. This will be my dessert. Only this time, I make a different flavor and a different consistency. See, that's the great thing about Eat-Smart: you can choose from two delicious flavors and add a wide variety of additional ingredients like fruits, sugar-free puddings, and even nuts, so you never get bored with them—and you can make them like a milk-shake or thicker, just like pudding.

This time I'm going to make the Chocolate-Chocolate Chip flavor into pudding. I simply add one scoop of the Eat-Smart powder into a small glass (actually, it's like a large, rounded coffee mug), then I add a very small amount of cold water. I mix it carefully with a spoon, until it turns into the creamy, thick consistency of pudding. The chocolate is my favorite for pudding, because it has real little chocolate chips in it. Boy, these are tasty, and they totally satisfy my sweet tooth.

I know I'm a little biased, because I work at the company that created them, but they're almost too good if you ask me… and I believe, *wholeheartedly*, in what we provide! In fact, after I tell my friends about them, and they try them, they often call or email me right away to tell me how much they love the flavors of Eat-Smart and that it tastes too good to be "good" for them. That makes me feel good—because we worked *really, really* hard to develop such a fantastically healthy and good-tasting supplement. (By the way, if you're interested in learning more, you can find Eat-Smart at many supplement retailers, like GNC (General Nutrition Centers, found nationwide), or online at iSatori.com/eatsmart).

Now, it's close to 10:00 p.m., so I sit down to review my notes from today and start planning for tomorrow. The next day, however, I won't be weight training; instead I will be doing cardiovascular exercise, so I really only have to plan my meals.

That's how I put all the basic pieces together. It's pretty simple and, best of all, it's worked well for me, and many, many others Daniel has helped, and I'm certain it can work just as well for you too. As you can plainly see, there is nothing overcomplicated about the workouts, eating smarter, nor the nutritional supplements I take. *There is no magic.* To be honest, once I learned all of this, I'd say most people make it way more complex, like I did, than it needs to be. Now, make no mistake about it, I'm not saying it's easy. Rather, I believe it's simple. It's simple to follow a plan like this, as long as you've carefully planned it out. But thankfully, all that is already done for you. The Daily Eating Journals and Workout Sheets are ready for you to download and start using. All you have to do is follow the steps, like I did.

TO CONCLUDE...

As you can see, putting the pieces together for Audrey was not all that complicated. However, over the course of my experience in working with ordinary people, making extraordinary transformations, two fundamental realities have become increasingly evident to me.

First, diets *never* work, for long-term success.

Second, if someone else can do it, that means others, like you, can do it too.

And the good news is, as we have learned from the stories of real people in this book, there is *always* hope, and it is never too late to change. *Never.*

So, it's time for your "Satori" moment, isn't it?

You bet.

And now that you have the answers to improve the way you look and feel, anything, and I mean *anything*, is possible.

Remember, we will be with you, along your journey, *every* step of the way! You can think of us as your "success coach!"

Until we meet again,

-Stephen Adelé

(AKA: Daniel Stephens)

DIETS SUCK!

Frequently Asked Questions

(After Reading the Book)

Q: This all sounds good, but does your program *really* work?

A: Yes! The proof can be found in the hundreds upon hundreds of successful transformation stories we have been a part of over the past 10 years. They provide real-world evidence that making lasting change, from the lessons we've shared in this book, is in fact possible. It doesn't matter if you're 25 or 75, overweight or just want to go from good to great in your physique, this program can work for anyone willing to follow it to the letter, just like the others before you. (And you can find their inspiring stories online at iSatori.com.)

Q: I am excited to get started—where should I begin?

A: First, I'd go online and join our lively, supportive community at iSatori.com; then sign up to start the 7-step program that will take you through each of the seven lessons from this book. Next, I'd find a "success coach" within our community to help keep you accountable and answer any questions, and pick up some Eat-Smart® shakes and bars. (Double Vanilla Ice Cream is my favorite flavored shake, and the Frosted Cinnamon Caramel Crunch are my favorite bars.) Then, please do me a huge favor, and drop me a quick note, on my personal Facebook (or Instagram) page, to let me know you've committed yourself to a new way of living… to a healthier, happier, and richer life. You can do that at facebook.com/stephenadele. I can't wait to hear from you!

Q: Are the transformation stories true, and are their photos real?

A: Absolutely! They are 100% real people, real stories, and unretouched, real photos. While some of the names of the characters in the main story of the book have been changed, the success stories presented in each Lesson are real, and we asked their permission to use their real names so we could share their stories, and pictures, in an authentic portrayal. Honestly, I couldn't live with myself if, in any way, I was trying to play tricks by falsifying their stories or pictures (that's just not the way I was raised).

Q: I'd like to join the same online community as Audrey found; where can I do that?

A: It's easy! Just come visit us at www.iSatori.com. Or, you can find me, and others from our team, on Facebook.com/iSatoriTech or Instagram. com/iSatori_Inc. To get the most out of your experience with us, and to optimize your results, I highly suggest you click on the "find a success coach" button and let us help you along your transformation journey.

Q: Why do I need to work out to lose weight?

A: There are more than a few reasons you should work out to lose weight, as well as countless "health" reasons to do so. First, and most important, working out will help you lose weight, faster. When you exercise, whether it's cardiovascular or resistance weight-training, you're revving up your body's metabolism (the rate our bodies burn calories). When you perform resistance weight training, you develop fresh, new lean muscle. Muscle is "metabolically active," meaning, unlike body fat that just sits there taking up space, muscle actually requires energy (or calories) to preserve and thereby turns your body into a 24/7 calorie-burning machine. Third, exercise on a regular basis helps regulate your body's blood/sugar (glucose) levels, so it helps control hunger cravings that can lead to unnecessary and destructive eating. And finally, building muscle is the *only* thing that can truly reshape your body—trading in unhealthy body fat for lean, shapely muscle.

Aside from that, and equally important, there are a generous number of reasons based on the latest scientific findings which show exercise can also improve many other health markers, such as lowering blood pressure, improving cognitive functions, strengthening the immune system, and fortifying our skeletal system, so our bones are stronger and more resilient. And the good news is, it actually takes only a small amount of physical activity to enjoy all of these wonderful, life-improving benefits!

Q: Where do I find more of the workout and eating worksheets?

A: You can find them online at www.iSatori.com in the *Diets Suck!* resources. There, you'll find the "basic" workout and eating journal sheets (the same ones you read in the book). And, as a bonus, we have also included other workouts and their journal sheets. Workouts that produce similar results, but vary in time, types of exercises, and advancement levels.

Q: Should I join a gym or work out from home?

A: I always answer this question the same. Go wherever you *will* work out and where you feel *most* comfortable. Whether that's at a commercial gym, at home with your own equipment, or at a studio gym with a personal trainer. There is no right or wrong way to work out, really. Personally, I like to change it up and spend a few weeks at a commercial gym and another couple of weeks working out at my home gym. And, of course, whenever I'm rushed, using my home gym is quite convenient and ensures I don't miss a valuable workout.

Q: Where can I find a qualified personal trainer?

A: Good question. There are lots of personal trainers out there, but not all of them are the same. Overall, though, using a personal trainer can be a great tool to help motive you, keep you accountable, and help you understand proper form and exercise technique. I suggest you do a little homework before selecting a personal trainer. You want to make sure they are certified from a reputable organization; and they have been a trainer for at least three years; and they train clients similar to you and your goals. A good place to start your search is online, where you can find a certified personal trainer in your area. Here are a couple of the organizations I trust, so you can locate your nearest certified personal trainer:

ACSM—American College of Sports Medicine

Web: certification.acsm.org/pro-finder

NSCA—National Strength and Conditioning Association

Web: www.nsca-lift.org (click "Personal Trainer" in the menu on the right and then click "Find a Personal Trainer" in the center column.)

If you can't locate one, please give us a call, and we'll help you find one. (We know lots of really good personal trainers.) You can reach us at 1-866-688-7679 or info@isatori.com.

Q: Why do you suggest using Eat-Smart in replacement of meals?

A: Let me first say you don't need to use supplements to achieve a transformation. I know this might sound funny coming from the owner of a supplement company. But the truth is, supplements are a "tool"—that's the way I promote using them—but I think you can find supplements to be a very useful way to help you reach your goals, faster and more conveniently. Eat-Smart meal-replacement protein shakes or bars, for example, are a very convenient (*and tasty*) way to substitute what could potentially be an unhealthy meal, or time-consuming or costly preparation of a meal, for a healthy, delicious "meal" that can be prepared in less than one minute and costs less than three dollars. Where else can you find the "perfect meal" for that little? Many of our most successful clients have found Eat-Smart to be a great way to take the guesswork out of eating healthy and ensuring you don't miss any meals during the day either, because we're all so darn busy. I know for me, personally, I use Eat-Smart about two or three times a day, and now that my taste buds are addicted, and my body loves them, I couldn't imagine life (and eating) any other way!

Q: What makes your Eat-Smart bar so different from the other protein bars out there?

A: Good question! Something to keep in mind, which we used as our guide in developing the Eat-Smart bar, was that we felt it was just as important what *wasn't* put into our bar as what *was* put into our bar. That is, if you look at our ingredients, we didn't add any worthless or unhealthy ingredients like aspartame, high fructose corn syrups, trans fats, gelatin proteins, and we kept the sugar alcohols very low. Equally important, we included high-quality, healthy ingredients like whey protein hydrolysates (the purest and most superior form of protein), natural flavors, fiber, vitamins and minerals. As you can see, there is a difference. We didn't cut any corners in its development, nor did we compromise on any ingredients at your expense. Yet, we made it taste delicious (the Chocolate Peanut Caramel Crunch tastes just like a rice crisp bar, dipped in chocolate). I have a hunch, after you try them, your body, and taste buds, will appreciate those differences too.

Q: I read you give away free bars to a children's charity for every purchase someone makes of Eat-Smart bars. Is that true?

A: Yes, it is true! When I was a kid, my Mom and I relied on the local food bank to eat. Now that I've been blessed to be in a positive position to "give back," I thought this was something I could really get behind and pour my heart into. So now, you can feel good about every purchase of Eat-Smart you make, because for every box of bars purchased, we donate an Eat-Smart bar to the "back-pack" program for hungry kids and their Feeding America initiative through the local food bank.

Sadly, there are over 16 million children who go home to empty cupboards every night after school. This program provides a back-pack full of food, every Friday afternoon, for kids to take home and provides them with nourishment and food over the weekend. There's nothing more rewarding than when we drop off hundreds of Eat-Smart bars to our local food bank, knowing we're supplying kids with a healthy, nutritious meal to eat. As you can imagine, it's a terrific cause I feel strongly about supporting.

Q: Where is the best place to find Eat-Smart products?

A: There are plenty of places you can find Eat-Smart products, but one of our favorite retailers, who carry pretty much everything from iSatori, is GNC. GNC, General Nutrition Centers, are conveniently located nationwide or online. You can also find Eat-Smart and other iSatori products online at Drugstore.com. If you can't find what you're looking for, or want to get personalized service with your purchases, please visit us directly at iSatori.com or by calling us at 1-866-688-7679.

Q: What should I do if I've slipped up and fallen off the wagon?

A: First of all, take a moment to realize *everyone* slips up, including and especially me. All of our success stories did. It's inevitable we all will, at some point in time. The key is not to let a slip up derail you from the great work you've put into your program so far. If you've missed a workout, skipped a meal, or ate poorly, don't allow yourself to get stressed out. Simply pick up where you left off and get yourself back on track. Schedule your next workout. Prepare your next healthy meal. Remember, it's important that you focus on progress and not perfection. It's the consistency of your new, improved approach to life and eating that will win over time, *every time*, and produce the extraordinary transformation you deserve.

Q: What should I do if I'm hungry, but it's not time to eat?

A: If you're hungry, yet it's not time to eat… eat anyway. *That's right.* Rather than starve yourself or deprive yourself (that's what typical fad diets do), go ahead and eat your next meal or shake or bar. Listening to your body, and not fighting against it, is essential in learning to improve your lifestyle and change the relationship you have with food and your body. One thing to consider, however, is that if you are continually hungry, my hunch is, you're not eating *enough* at each meal. Try slightly increasing the amount of protein you consume at each meal, and consider whether that helps alleviate any hunger issues you might be experiencing.

Q: Is alcohol off limits?

A: No. While beer and hard liquor is "off limits"—because they contain far too many sugars and calories—a glass of red wine a couple of times a week is perfectly acceptable. Reason is, red wine contains a natural phytosterol, from the grape skins found in red wine, called resveratrol. You can think of resveratrol as a healthy antioxidant and something that, according to the most recent scientific evidence, may help us live longer by protecting the "good cells" in the body.

Q: Are there any dietary supplements you recommend for aiding in weight loss?

A: Yes, indeed. But you need to be careful—there are a lot of hucksters out there, selling weight-loss supplements that have little to no evidence they will be effective or safe. Weight-loss supplements that have ample scientific evidence, and ones I trust, are: green tea (look for extracts high in EGCG), conjugated linoleic acid (otherwise known as CLA), 7-Keto, green coffee bean (look for at least 60% chlorogenic acid content), yerba mate, and L-carnitine. If you can handle the stimulant effect, caffeine (or guarana, the herbal equivalent of caffeine) is proven to help the body use more calories as energy, through a process called thermogenesis. Remember, these weight-loss supplements are just that—a "supplemental tool" to help you in your efforts to lose weight, faster. They should always be used as a part of an overall lifestyle improvement program, consisting of exercise and eating smart. And when considering any supplements, you should check with your doctor first, to make sure you are in good health, before using them. If you want more information on any of these types of weight-loss ingredients, or other supplements, you can visit some great resourceful websites called **ultimatefatburner.com** or **supplementreviews.com**, where you can find unbiased and expert reviews on any type of nutritional supplements available, including the ones I just mentioned.

Q: What other supplements did Audrey use?

A: Aside from using Eat-Smart religiously as her "meal replacement," Audrey also uses several other supplements she finds helpful. Those supplements she uses daily are *a multi-vitamin/mineral* formula (GNC Vita-pack ultra-mega woman's brand) as a health "insurance policy"; *calcium* (citrate form is better) for stronger bones; Vitamin D3, because it has so much positive research for women, with much of it pertaining to cancer; *probiotics*, to help with gut and intestinal health; and a *fiber drink* (like Metamucil) at night. These are what you would consider "health" supplements; whereas, she also takes other "performance" related supplements, around her workouts, such as *Restoraid*, an amino acid/electrolyte recovery drink by our company, iSatori, that is sipped on (using a shaker bottle) during workouts to help reduce any muscle soreness and recover faster after workouts; as well as *gcbLEAN800*, a "stimulant-free" weight-loss supplement that combines green coffee bean and raspberry ketones. Along with these supplements, Audrey is sure to drink at least 8 to 10 glasses of water, daily, to ensure she is well hydrated. Always be sure to check with your doctor prior to starting any supplement or exercise program.

Q: I started making great progress with my weight loss, but then I "hit a wall," and it stopped; what should I do?

A: First of all, don't give up hope. You can do this. Sometimes our bodies just take a little longer and resist our desire to lose weight. If this happens, here's what you can try. Your body may be resisting the weight loss because of a buildup of toxins, and you many need to "detox." Nothing extreme, just a simple three-day detox, whereby a cleansing effect should do the trick to help "unlock" the substances that might be holding back your weight-loss progress. For the three-day detox, I suggest you follow the plan at iSatori.com in the *Diets Suck!* resources. *It's easy*—all you need is a blender and a few fresh grocery items.

Q: Your program is working great for me, and I don't want it to end. What can I do to make sure it keeps working?

A: Congratulations is in order first! But remember, it's not the "program" that is working—it's *you* who is working, perfectly! All you need to do is adopt the mindset that this isn't a short-term "diet," and your new ways of eating, exercising, and thinking about yourself are permanent lifestyle changes that should last a lifetime. Another great way to keep your progress going strong is to help other people do the same and help them follow in your footsteps. By continually practicing what you preach, you'll be more inclined to carry out your new approach to living through "leading by example."

Q: How can I share this book with someone I care about, without offending them?

A: Great question. Obviously, we need to be mindful about how we share this book with those we love and care about. First, though, it's important you keep in mind, by sharing this book, you're doing something very important, and frankly, something that could positively change someone's life forever. One way to do this might be to purchase a copy of *Diets Suck!* for someone, and give it to them or mail it to them, and compliment it with a handwritten card. Taking the time to write out a card shows them just how much you care. The card could say something like this… *"Dear _____, I just finished reading this great new book. Not only did I find it an easy read, but it was full of inspiring and interesting stories that really struck home. I think you'll enjoy reading this book as much as I did. Please let me know what you think of it, once you're done. With Love, _____!"* I'm fairly certain this approach to sharing a copy of the *Diets Suck!* book will come across the way you intend—with plenty of love and care.

Q: If I want to get a hold of you because I have more questions, or need additional information, how can I do that?

A: There are plenty of ways to get a hold of me, or anyone at my company, who will be glad to help. You can reach me personally at Facebook.com/stephenadele. (I may take a little while to get back to you, but I will, I promise.) You can find our company, including me, online anytime, at our Facebook.com/iSatoriTech or Instagram.com/iSatori_Inc pages; by emailing us at info@isatori.com; or if you prefer to talk to one of our qualified professionals, call us toll-free at 1-866-688-7679. We're always available to help you in any way we can.

P.S. Before we let this opportunity slip away from us… I would be remiss if I didn't bring this up to you. That is, the greatest tragedy of reading this book would be that you choose to close it, put it away on the bookshelf, and never do anything with it. *Let's not let that happen.* Instead, let's focus on getting you from where you are today to where you want to be… to transform your body *and* your life. After all, that is what you truly deserve. So, do yourself a favor. Hop online and join our lively, supportive community at isatori.com; sign up to start the 7-step Eat-Smart transformation program; and email me to let me know you've committed yourself to a new way of living… to a healthier, happier, and richer life. I can't wait to hear from you! ☺

You Now	Who You Want to Be

**JOIN ME AT ISATORI.COM AND
GET YOUR <u>FREE</u> SPECIAL REPORTS**

(With my compliments, as our way of saying thanks!)

DIETS SUCK!

Sample Upper Body Workout Sheet

Name: Audrey	Date: June 7th	Start Time: 12:40	Stop Time: 1:05
		Estimated Time: 25 minutes	Total Time: 25 minutes

GROUP	EXERCISE	WEIGHT (POUNDS)	GOAL REPS	ACTUAL
Chest	Bench press	55	15–20	16
		65	12	12
		65	10	9
		75	8	8
		75	8	8
Back	Lat pull downs	40	15–20	15
		50	12	12
		60	10	11
		70	8	8
		70	8	8
Shoulders	Seated dumbbell side lateral raises	5	15–20	18
		10	12	12
		10	10	10
		15	8	8
		15	8	6
Biceps	Preacher curl machine	25	15–20	20
		35	12	12
		45	10	10
		55	8	8
		55	8	8
Triceps	Assisted bar dips (Bodyweight with band assist)	with band assist	15–20	15
		with band assist	12	12
		with band assist	10	10
		with band assist	8	8
		with band assist	8	6

Visit isatori.com in the *Diets Suck!* resources for more blank worksheets.

Perform each exercise once with no rest between; after finishing one "Giant Set," take 60 seconds, get a drink of water, stretch, or focus on your breathing and then start from the top and perform every exercise again. Each time you go through a Giant Set, increase the weight while decreasing the number of reps. Repeat until all five Giant Sets have been completed.

Now, pick your favorite cardiovascular exercise machine, set the timer for 20 minutes, and use a high enough intensity level to make it difficult but not impossible to perform.

For full explanations and to watch each workout in progress, along with our personal tips and tricks, please come visit our online video channel at www.YouTube.com/iSatoriTech. Here, you can watch us take you through each and every exercise, as well as highlight our favorite cardio exercises. We also share with you our most popular easy-to-prepare, hunger-smashing, protein-packed meals.

DIETS SUCK!

Sample Lower Body Workout Sheet

Name: Audrey	Date: June 9th	Start Time: 12:37	Stop Time: 1:00
		Estimated Time: 25 minutes	Total Time: 23 minutes

GROUP	EXERCISE	WEIGHT (POUNDS)	GOAL REPS	ACTUAL
Quadriceps (front of leg)	Squats	55	15–20	15
		65	12	12
		75	10	10
		85	8	8
		85	8	9
Quadriceps (front of leg)	Leg extensions	40	15–20	18
		35	12	12
		45	10	10
		50	8	8
		50	8	8
Hamstrings (back of leg)	Leg curl	35	15–20	16
		40	12	12
		45	10	10
		50	8	8
		50	8	8
Calves	Calf raises on Hack Squat	+70	15–20	20
		+80	12	12
		+80	10	10
		+90	8	8
		+90	8	10
Abdominals (stomach)	Seated Crunches (on machine)	10	20	25
		20	15	15
		30	12	15
		30	12	12
		30	12	12

Visit iSatori.com in the *Diets Suck!* resources for more blank worksheets.

DIETS SUCK!

Daily Nutritional Planning Sheet

Date: _____ Day of the Week: _____ Activity Level (1-5): _____

*If you use an Eat-Smart protein nutrition shake or Eat-Smart bar in replace of a meal, simply write it out within the "Protein" line.

Meal #1   Time: _____
Protein: _____
Carb: _____
Veggies: _____
Drink: _____

Meal #2 (Snack)   Time: _____
Protein: _____
Carb: _____
Veggies: _____
Drink: _____

Meal #3   Time: _____
Protein: _____
Carb: _____
Veggies: _____
Drink: _____

Meal #4 (Snack)   Time: _____
Protein: _____
Carb: _____
Veggies: _____
Drink: _____

Meal #5   Time: _____
Protein: _____
Carb: _____
Veggies: _____
Drink: _____

Visit iSatori.com in the *Diets Suck!* resources for more blank worksheets.

DIETS SUCK!

Your First 12 Weeks

Name:			Goal:				

Week	Sunday	Monday	Tuesday	Wednesday	Thursday	Friday	Saturday
1	DATE: OFF	DATE: UPPER BODY Workout #1	DATE: CARDIO Workout #2	DATE: LOWER BODY Workout #3	DATE: CARDIO Workout #4	DATE: UPPER BODY Workout #5	DATE: CARDIO Workout #6
2	DATE: OFF	DATE: LOWER BODY Workout #7	DATE: CARDIO Workout #8	DATE: UPPER BODY Workout #9	DATE: CARDIO Workout #10	DATE: LOWER BODY Workout #11	DATE: CARDIO Workout #12
3	DATE: OFF	DATE: UPPER BODY Workout #13	DATE: CARDIO Workout #14	DATE: LOWER BODY Workout #15	DATE: CARDIO Workout #16	DATE: UPPER BODY Workout #17	DATE: CARDIO Workout #18
4	DATE: OFF	DATE: LOWER BODY Workout #19	DATE: CARDIO Workout #20	DATE: UPPER BODY Workout #21	DATE: CARDIO Workout #22	DATE: LOWER BODY Workout #23	DATE: CARDIO Workout #24
5	DATE: OFF	DATE: UPPER BODY Workout #25	DATE: CARDIO Workout #26	DATE: LOWER BODY Workout #27	DATE: CARDIO Workout #28	DATE: UPPER BODY Workout #29	DATE: CARDIO Workout #30
6	DATE: OFF	DATE: LOWER BODY Workout #31	DATE: CARDIO Workout #32	DATE: UPPER BODY Workout #33	DATE: CARDIO Workout #34	DATE: LOWER BODY Workout #35	DATE: CARDIO Workout #36
7	DATE: OFF	DATE: UPPER BODY Workout #37	DATE: CARDIO Workout #38	DATE: LOWER BODY Workout #39	DATE: CARDIO Workout #40	DATE: UPPER BODY Workout #41	DATE: CARDIO Workout #42
8	DATE: OFF	DATE: LOWER BODY Workout #43	DATE: CARDIO Workout #44	DATE: UPPER BODY Workout #45	DATE: CARDIO Workout #46	DATE: LOWER BODY Workout #47	DATE: CARDIO Workout #48
9	DATE: OFF	DATE: UPPER BODY Workout #49	DATE: CARDIO Workout #50	DATE: LOWER BODY Workout #51	DATE: CARDIO Workout #52	DATE: UPPER BODY Workout #53	DATE: CARDIO Workout #54
10	DATE: OFF	DATE: LOWER BODY Workout #55	DATE: CARDIO Workout #56	DATE: UPPER BODY Workout #57	DATE: CARDIO Workout #58	DATE: LOWER BODY Workout #59	DATE: CARDIO Workout #60
11	DATE: OFF	DATE: UPPER BODY Workout #61	DATE: CARDIO Workout #62	DATE: LOWER BODY Workout #63	DATE: CARDIO Workout #64	DATE: UPPER BODY Workout #65	DATE: CARDIO Workout #66
12	DATE: OFF	DATE: LOWER BODY Workout #67	DATE: CARDIO Workout #68	DATE: UPPER BODY Workout #69	DATE: CARDIO Workout #70	DATE: LOWER BODY Workout #71	DATE: CARDIO Workout #72

DIETS SUCK!

Upper Body Workout Sheet

Name:	Date:	Start Time:	Stop Time:
		Estimated Time:	Total Time:

GROUP	EXERCISE	WEIGHT (POUNDS)	GOAL REPS	ACTUAL
Chest				
Back				
Shoulders				
Biceps				
Triceps				

Visit iSatori.com in the *Diets Suck!* resources for more blank worksheets.

DIETS SUCK!

Lower Body Workout Sheet

Name:	Date:	Start Time:	Stop Time:
		Estimated Time:	Total Time:

GROUP	EXERCISE	WEIGHT (POUNDS)	GOAL REPS	ACTUAL
Quadriceps (front of leg)				
Quadriceps (front of leg)				
Hamstrings (back of leg)				
Calves				
Abdominals (stomach)				

Visit iSatori.com in the *Diets Suck!* resources for more blank worksheets.

GRATITUDE

In life, success can be measured in many ways. For me, I've always measured my personal success by the quality of enduring and loving relationships. And, professionally, by the number of lives I am able to positively impact as a result of my work. So, to be quite frank, I feel very successful. Yet, success does not happen in isolation. And this book was no exception.

With that said, I would like to extend my deepest gratitude to all those whose contributions to this book made it a success:

First, to my loving family—for teaching me the most important lessons in life, every day, and for keeping the lights on at night, so I could stay up writing; my mother and father, who thankfully taught me early on to value family above all else and to lead with my heart; and my Grandmother Audrey for teaching me how to believe in myself and continually stressing the importance of communication through writing.

Then, there were those "behind the scenes" friends, clients, and co-workers who are equally responsible for the creation of this book. I am eternally grateful for their support. (May the Universal Law reward you tenfold!) These wonderful people are:

Sue Mosebar, for the magic that was created the day we first talked about writing this book and for continuing to make it better and better along the way; and, it goes without saying, for your incredible editing skills; Andrea Clem, for providing us the "spark" to tell your incredibly inspiring story by choosing to live by example for all of us at iSatori and whose story will inspire so many others to walk in your footsteps; Albert Rivera, Kay Evans, Kim Bowser, Carla Iansiti, Tony Martinez, and Shari "Fitness" Friedman, for allowing us to share your truly inspirational stories, for once again reminding me why I love what I do so much, and for continually encouraging others to see how great life can be when you transform your life and live as you have; all the team members at iSatori, for making work so much fun and letting me include your cameos in our book; the Phillips family—Bill, Shawn, Shelly, and especially BP, for the educational experience you provided me (BP, you are deeply missed); David Sandler, for your expert advice and insight into the "workouts"; Brian Harvat, for so eloquently laying out this book, from cover to cover—I love your creativity and the passion you put into your work; Rich Wysockey and Brett Seeley, for your engaging photographs found throughout our website and within our book; my dearest Vistage Group friends, for teaching me the discipline to "finish what I start"; Kenneth Gillett, for believing enough in our "little" project to pour your heart and expertise into bringing it to market; Dr. Andrew Rosenthal, for trusting enough in me to lend your name to our project and for your many contributions along my journey; and to Charles Atlas and his funny little cartoon advertisement, found in most comic books, who originally inspired me to build my best body.

And most of all, I'd like to thank you, the reader of this book, for investing your precious time in me and for trusting that I will guide you on the right path. Thank you.

DIETS SUCK!

7 LESSONS TO YOUR OWN
PHYSICAL & EMOTIONAL TRANSFORMATION

LESSON #1: FIND A SUPPORT SYSTEM

You must find truly caring and compassionate support to help encourage and reinforce your positive lifestyle changes.

LESSON #2: KNOW YOUR WHY

Unlock your reasons, and know your why, to draw you toward your transformation goals.

LESSON #3: SET A SMART GOAL

Think big, but start small: set big, SMART, long-term transformation goals!

LESSON #4: ACCEPT YOURSELF

You must know, accept, and *love* your body, as it is.

LESSON #5: LOOK INWARD

To help guide your transformation journey to lasting weight loss, you must no longer look outward and instead look inward.

LESSON #6: GET MOVING (AND STAY MOVING)

Consistency, when it comes to working out and losing weight, wins over time, every time.

LESSON #7: MAKE A COMMITMENT

Accept that it's not my fault I didn't eat right and work out. Today is the day I have *committed* to make a permanent change, and through my very own successful transformation, will *help others* around me to walk in my footsteps.